O.XI. 48

THE VANISHING TRIBES OF KENYA

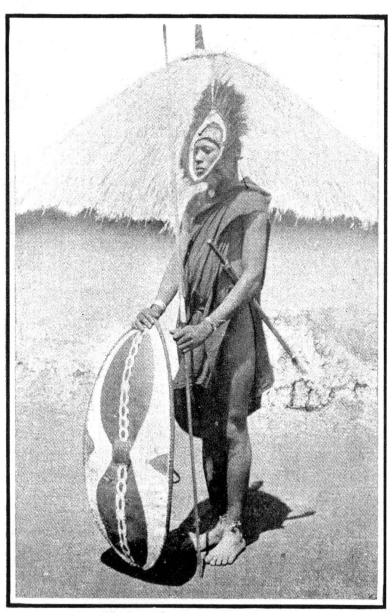

Mwimbe Warrior in Full Dress.

The weapons and headdress are simply a copy of the Masai Morans dress.

THE

VANISHING
TRIBES OF KENYA

A DESCRIPTION OF THE MANNERS & CUSTOMS OF THE
PRIMITIVE & INTERESTING TRIBES DWELLING ON
THE VAST SOUTHERN SLOPES OF MOUNT
KENYA, & THEIR FAST DISAPPEARING
NATIVE METHODS OF LIFE

BY

Major G. St J. ORDE BROWNE, O.B.E.(Mil.)

F.R.G.S., F.R.A.I., F.Z.S.

*Late Royal Artillery, Senior Commissioner, Tanganyika, Fellow of the
American Geographical Society, Membre de l'Institut
d'Anthropologie Suisse, &c.*

WITH MANY ILLUSTRATIONS & 2 MAPS

London
Seeley, Service & Co. Limited
196 Shaftesbury Avenue
1925

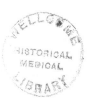
PRINTED IN GREAT BRITAIN BY THE
RIVERSIDE PRESS LIMITED, EDINBURGH

INTRODUCTION

THIS book is an effort to record the writer's observations of the manners and customs of a primitive and interesting group of tribes who dwell on the southern slopes of Mount Kenya. Development in that part of Africa is proceeding so rapidly that it is important to describe as much as possible of the fast-disappearing native methods of life; even since the accompanying notes and photographs were taken changes have taken place and much has already vanished for ever. Since the various tribes with which this book deals are small in number and limited in area, it is obvious that their own peculiar customs can have little chance of survival in the face of the general intermixture of tribes taking place under European administration.

A considerable quantity of literature already exists, dealing with the more important peoples of this region; the Akikuyu have been fairly fully dealt with, while some records also exist of the Akamba; the Meru of North-East Kenya have also been studied to some extent, though much still remains to be done. The philology of the region has been adequately examined, and the local languages and dialects are definitely placed.

Between these various peoples, however, there comes a debatable region, inhabited by a group of small tribes possessing many of the characteristics of their neighbours, but also retaining numerous local peculiarities; and a study of these serves to reveal a wealth of most interesting detail, much of which seems to

5

Introduction

throw light upon that obscure subject—the migrations and early history of the Central African tribes. This book represents an effort to record such details before it is too late to observe them.

The observations and photographs were collected during some seven years, when I was very favourably situated for such a purpose; an astonishing amount of work was involved, and much patience was necessary; again and again notes had to be revised or rewritten, and descriptions altered in the light of further information. The illustrations are the survivors of an immense number of pictures taken, the bulk of which proved to be failures. It is no easy task to take a photograph of a ceremony, surrounded by several hundred excited natives, with the air laden with dust, and the light probably quite unfavourable; much patience is also necessary to win the confidence of the people sufficiently to allow one to witness and record the various performances. This must be my excuse for the limitations of my work (handicapped also, as it was, by an interlude of some years' war service) and my failure to secure many interesting details. I have throughout tried to record only the results of personal observation and investigation, and I have preferred to leave a question untouched rather than fill in the gap with plausible or picturesque accounts which I could not actually verify. I am aware that in some directions my descriptions or suggestions may conflict with those of other observers better qualified than myself to analyse or explain native customs. I am content to put down my own results and to leave them as a small contribution of material for the study of the great science of Ethnology.

The years during which this work was done (1909-1916) were exceptionally favourable, for they saw the change from practically untouched primitive con-

Introduction

ditions to the establishment of definite European administration. During this time I was stationed as Assistant Commissioner at various Government posts in the area in question, and was intimately concerned in the construction work of government. Resources were very limited, and we had neither the wish nor the ability to progress by means of military action; so a comprehension of the native outlook and mentality was essential for any success. With no troops within a hundred miles, and a couple of dozen native police as one's only effective force, there was certainly little chance of overawing or intimidating the many thousands of natives all around, so one was entirely dependent upon some knowledge of the people for any success in one's work.

In order to get into contact with such shy and suspicious folk it was necessary to resort to all sorts of expedients, and at times one's camp had a strong suggestion of a circus: magic lanterns, conjuring tricks, and fireworks, all served to attract the natives to begin with, and, later, to impress them with the power and mystery of European knowledge; the ever-useful medicine chest was even more valuable in securing friends, though less striking and impressive at first sight. Such expedients may seem a somewhat cheap and undignified introduction, but it must be remembered that one was dealing with people who were very like children, and who responded to the same methods of approach; perhaps some people would have advocated the machine-gun and the lash as a means of attracting attention and establishing authority. Be that as it may, we pursued mainly methods of peaceful penetration, with a corresponding economy in lives and expenditure. The present book is the result of some years of living under such conditions.

In collecting records of this nature there is always

Introduction

a danger of accepting the information most readily offered; and even when the more obvious mistakes of this nature have been avoided there still remains an instinctive tendency to rely upon some quick and intelligent informant, rather than on an older and stupider person who is, nevertheless, probably more accurate and reliable. I found by practical experience that it was more satisfactory to get one's facts and details from the less promising informants rather than to collect with ease a large amount of notes which had subsequently to be drastically revised when checked with results from another native. Old men are usually reliable but reticent. I obtained much information from them, however, by means of contradictions—that is to say, I would start by the statement that I knew all about the matter with which I was dealing; I would then tell them what I knew, embroidering this with invented details, with the result that I was met, first with a superior smile, and then with a denial and a correction. In this way I was able to elaborate and check my accounts of the various ceremonies. Old women were also valuable, once they could be induced to start, for they are the best repositories of folk-stories and anecdotes. The friendly and intelligent young man, however, with his ready flow of information, has, despite his good intentions, proved a trap for many guileless investigators.

The native's ignorance of grammar is a great handicap. He fails to grasp that the pronoun " you " need not necessarily mean the person addressed with his own personality. One has, therefore, to be careful to keep the difference between " you " and " a man " quite clear; in fact it is usually best to acknowledge the concrete outlook, and accept the fact that the speaker is always describing his own actions in his position as, say, a warrior, and that he finds it very difficult to grasp

Introduction

the conditions suggested by such a preface as " supposing you were an old man." I found it a great help to use a set of little cardboard figures, cut out and painted to represent the various members of a family; these could be moved about the table, so as to meet each other, give the customary greetings, quarrel, arrange a marriage, and so forth—their words in each case being spoken by a selected person among the spectators. This sort of marionette play seemed to make it much easier for all concerned to describe the dialogues and actions, and I frequently went through lengthy and dramatic scenes, with a dozen or more figures and quite a village of paper huts. I was at first uneasy lest some magic effect might be suspected or feared, but I never found that this difficulty arose.

In the case of very many natives I was the first white man to whom they had ever spoken; often the women or the old men would say that they had never even seen a European, when I visited a remote village. This made them shy on first acquaintance, but much more friendly and confiding subsequently, so that I had little difficulty in persuading them to let me witness various functions which I was afterwards surprised to find jealously guarded from European eyes among much more sophisticated natives.

The rate of progress was astonishing. Communities among which the war-horn and the poisoned arrow were quite the possible form of greeting were five years later thoroughly used to Europeans, buying and selling in coin, going away to work, and using piece goods, steel tools and matches as if they had known them all their lives. I have seen an Indian shop doing a thriving trade in a village where only a year or two previously I had bartered a handful of salt for a chicken; and I have heard a native complain of the quality of a box of matches when he still had hanging

Introduction

in his hut his quiver with a fire-stick and block tied to it.[1]

Such rapid change has naturally meant the disappearance of many old customs. The smaller tribes are all fast becoming merged in their larger and more important neighbours, while every influence tends to make the young people despise and forget the old traditions. In 1918 I revisited Embu, and asked about certain dances and customs which I had seen and recorded only six or eight years earlier. I was in some cases told that they had already been abandoned and forgotten.

My book has little to do with the system of administration or the work of the officers who established it. I have dealt with the natives themselves, and have tried to keep the personal element in the background.

My thanks are due, for assistance in checking various details, to Messrs Kenyon-Slaney, R. G. Stone, and the late Mr W. C. Allen, all of the Kenya Administration, also to various other helpers, European and African.

---

[1] A very apt description of society in the barter stage, which exactly fits the above stage, is to be found in Adam Smith's *Wealth of Nations*, ch. iv.

CONTENTS

Contents

LIST OF ILLUSTRATIONS

13

List of Illustrations

Maps

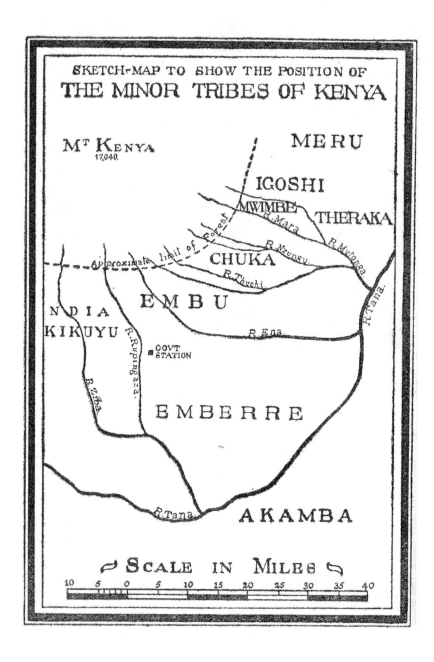

SKETCH-MAP TO SHOW THE POSITION OF
THE MINOR TRIBES OF KENYA

THE VANISHING TRIBES
OF KENYA

CHAPTER I

HISTORY

THE early history of the southern and eastern portions of Mount Kenya would appear to be closely connected with the geography of the country—that is to say, all the movements of the natives in that region seem to have depended mainly on climatic and geographical conditions. It must be borne in mind that no records worth the name exist at all, and that such oral tradition as is to be found is scanty and vague in the extreme. There can be little doubt, however, that the state of affairs existing at the advent of European influence was a new and unsettled one; probably within what would be, in European history, comparatively recent times, an entirely different state of affairs existed to that found by the first white explorers.

The main factor in the development of the country has been the great peak of Kenya, with its dominating effect upon the whole nature of the region. The equable climate, the even and reliable rainfall, the

History

richness of the soil, and the existence of the forest belt, all result from the presence of the great extinct volcano. A proper appreciation of conditions, both old and new, can only be realized, therefore, by a constant recollection of the natural features which must always have played a leading part in the history of the country.

Rising at its summit to 17,000 feet, Mount Kenya stands isolated on all sides from any neighbouring heights by a wide plain, which averages some 5000 feet above sea-level. About forty miles to the west lie the Aberdares, a long chain which, though inferior in height to Kenya, still includes several peaks of over 12,000 feet. South and south-east, Kenya slopes down into the rolling plains of the Tana river, the latter forming the channel by which all the water from the southern slopes of the mountain is drained away. This river curves around the mountain at an average distance of some forty miles, until it turns towards the coast through the Mumoni Range. It forms a natural boundary to Kenya Province and its tribes, and serves as an effectual barrier between the Akikuyu with the allied tribes, and the Akamba on the other side of the Tana, though by no means preventing all intercourse. The slopes of Kenya, which are abrupt and well defined nearer the summit, fade gradually into the plain of the Tana, which at its lowest point is only some 2000 feet above sea-level.

This formation naturally leads to a great variety of

History

climate, vegetation and scenery; and it is doubtless owing to this great diversity that such differences are to be found among the tribes living upon the slopes of the mountain.

Below the snow-line there is an expanse of moor-like country, attractive in the rare intervals of sunshine, but usually enveloped in wet mists; this gradually merges into the bamboos which form a belt almost all round the mountain; these in turn give place to the dense virgin forest which covers the lower slopes until it meets the point at which human requirements have restricted it. It is this forest that plays so large a part in the development of the country. Climatically, it is presumably responsible for the occurrence of rain, while the soil reclaimed from it is of exceptional value for agriculture. From a more intimate point of view, it provided a safe refuge from any enemy that might attack a community living near its edge, while conversely, it afforded cover for raiding parties from another side of the mountain.

There is no doubt that the forest originally extended far beyond its present limits; even within the memory of living people it has been cut back to a surprising extent; on the northern slopes the forest belt has become very thin, and on the Aberdares, where the same action has been going on, there are places where the cultivated land almost reaches the bamboos, with no intervening forest proper at all.

On South-East Kenya, however, this process has been retarded. The forest belt is still fairly wide, while the country below it is far more wooded and uncultivated than is the case farther round the mountain. Still, there seems to be no doubt that there used to be a stretch of forest reaching far down into what are now the bare plains of the Tana.

From the scanty evidence to be obtained, it would appear that the present density of population is comparatively recent; all the native traditions indicate a state of change, almost of invasion, which created a need for the land around the base of the mountain among people pressing upwards from the less fertile plains.

Among all the minor tribes of Kenya the Chuka alone claim to have lived in their country from the beginning of things; other sections connect themselves with the Akamba, or give some other account of their early history which indicates an alien origin. All, however, agree in saying that they have steadily encroached on the forest, and that it did not originally belong to them; the view generally taken is that the present inhabitants were plain-dwellers, and that they overcame and exterminated the original forest people by weight of numbers rather than by force of arms. The Chuka, however, do not altogether admit this, though they agree in saying that there was a race which inhabited the forest in former times which is now extinct.

All accounts of this race seem to agree: they were small in stature—apparently some four feet six or so, as an average—they wore beards and were generally

History

hairy; they did no sort of agricultural work, but lived by hunting and bee-keeping; they lived in dug-out caves, ten or twelve to a hut; the ground apparently being hollowed out and then just roofed over to keep out the rain. They were cunning and diplomatic, but not war-like. There is some suggestion that they made pottery, but there seems to be no sort of concrete evidence to support this idea. No traces of any sort of habitation of such people seem to have been found, but no doubt such slight remains as there might be would be very hard to recognize now. There seems to be no sort of idea that they used any kind of stone implement; or that they drew any sort of picture like the bushman.

The above account seems at first sight to fit the present tribe of Wanderobo; it is noteworthy, however, that all sections agree in saying that the people described were not Wanderobo, or in any way connected with them. The two peoples are separated, and occupy quite different positions in the minds of the existing natives. The name generally given to this extinct race is " Agumba," though "Asi " is an alternative to be met with. It is said that these people were originally very numerous, but that they gradually dwindled away with the cutting of the forest — although on friendly terms with the invaders—until only a few old men were left. These old men then turned into the " Plantain Birds," which inhabit the forest to this day in large numbers, and they are to be heard talking their original language together in the forest at night.

History

It may be remarked that old men will generally attribute the ownership of the forest land to these people, and the regulations which govern the use of land seem to take this theory into account. Also, it is curious that the old custom dictated a red feather from one of these birds as an addition to the head-dress of a warrior when he had killed a man. No veneration is shown to these birds, and the Agumba seem to be rapidly fading from the memory of the people, in every detail.

Admitting the existence of these scattered and retiring people in the depths of the forest, there seem to have been three influences at work upon the southern and eastern sides of Kenya. These may be classified as: (1) a north-westerly invasion, or pressure, from across the Tana; (2) a south-westerly invasion from the north, via Meru; (3) a south-easterly invasion from the western side of the mountain.

This classification is entirely tentative, and it is impossible to produce much tangible evidence in support of it; it is merely offered as an explanation of the state of affairs found when European administration first appeared in the country. There can be little doubt that, at that time, Chuka was the centre of pressure from the quarters named.

It would seem that successive waves of immigrants gradually invaded the slopes of Kenya, and established themselves on the land reclaimed by burning the forest; as they came to appreciate the better climate and superior fertility of the upper country, they continued the movement upwards into the wooded slopes of the mountain, clearing it more or less thoroughly according to their numbers.

Here, again, the nature of the country plays a large part. In what is now the Kikuyu country, the slopes were gentle and uniform, and no great natural obstacles existed in the form of deep gorges or impassable rivers; the community, therefore, spread evenly up the heights, preserving communication with each other, and holding together as a tribe to a large extent; the very fact of the country being free of obstacles in itself served to knit them closer, since it rendered them all the more likely to be raided or attacked in force by their neighbours. The Akikuyu, therefore, remained as one community, with similar customs and the same language, with slight modifications. The whole of the plain between the Aberdares and Kenya became filled with the same agricultural and pastoral people, united by a common origin, and further kept together by the danger of a raid from their restless neighbours, the Masai.

Farther east, however, conditions were very different. The rivers ran in rocky gorges, whose timber-clad sides were swept with torrents of rain in the wet season, rendering all paths across them precarious and difficult. The nature of the ground made it much less desirable for cultivation, and a smaller number of people, therefore, occupied it, settling in isolated communities between the deep valleys of the river-beds, large tongues of forest being left along the less useful ridges, to accentuate still further the isolating effect of the valley.

In this way, Chuka, and, to a lesser extent, Embu and Mwimbe, came to be inhabited by an independent and wild set of natives, who became more and more unlike their neighbours as time went on. Each section isolated itself and formed its own customs—or preserved those lost elsewhere—without being affected by the little community living the other side of some almost impassable gorge.

This scantiness, too, of population, consequent upon the difficult nature of the country, must have rendered the absorption of the original population less complete. Presuming that some sort of people such as are described really occupied the forest, it is obvious that they must have largely affected the invaders, when the latter were not in overwhelming numbers. Apparently, therefore, the south-eastern slopes of Kenya became the stronghold of the most backward and primitive portion of the growing population of the country, chiefly owing to the character of the natural features: isolated among their forests and gorges, the inhabitants remained primitive and unprogressive, while the neighbouring Meru were establishing themselves in the north, and the Akikuyu were spreading over the plains to the south and west of Kenya. The more desirable country had also its disadvantages, and the Akikuyu found themselves assailed by the Masai, which must have tended to unite them in the face of the common enemy. The Meru, too, were engaged in struggles with the tribes to their north while the Akamba ranged restlessly over the wide arid plains of the Tana. On South-East Kenya, however, there was little necessity and few facilities for a wandering life of plunder. There was room enough for each man to till the plot that he considered necessary, and a primitive existence created the desire for few novelties or exotic luxuries; there was little or no trade, and therefore no incentive to avarice. There were undoubtedly occasional raids by various enemies, but these were sufficiently rare and difficult of execution to make their occurrence the exception rather than the rule.

So the earliest state of affairs that can be assumed with any probability is the existence of a backward nucleus in and about the country now known as Chuka, with the three outside influences pressing upon it from the west (the Akikuyu), the north (the Meru) and the south-east (the Akamba). As these three forces acted upon this nucleus, they influenced it to some extent, and gave rise to the various divisions which now exist. Thus, the Akamba influence created the Emberre, who might almost as well be termed akin to the Akamba as to the Akikuyu. The Embu owed most to the Akikuyu proper, who became less and less characteristic of their main body as they travelled east, until the Ndia Kikuyu, although still calling themselves Kikuyu, adopted many customs and altered their language, until they might almost be considered a separate branch of their tribe. Next to them, the Embu

History

represented the first of the definite " minor tribes."
The already appreciable differences between the Ndia
Kikuyu and their more orthodox brethren become
much emphasized. Language and customs differ more
and more, while the name " Kikuyu " is dropped, the
people calling themselves " Embu."

To the north the same process was taking place:
the Meru tribes merged gradually into their southern
neighbours, until it becomes very difficult to say where
the Meru really end. Divided among themselves into
many sections, they hardly admit of any definite test of
origin. The inhabitants of Mwimbe, however, would
deny that they were Meru, as would their neighbours
of the Igoji; but both sections are, nevertheless,
strongly impregnated with Meru customs and idioms.

Between these three sections—Embu, Emberre and
Mwimbe—there remain the Chuka.

It requires only a very cursory examination to see
that here we have the element that is responsible for
all the differences in the other minor tribes. Whatever
eccentricity is noticeable in any of their neighbours
is generally accentuated in the Chuka; any distinctive
custom to be found in the other sections is generally
far more elaborate and characteristic in Chuka; any
peculiarity which is being given up by the Embu, or
the Mwimbe, usually turns out to be the established
Chuka custom. There are various details in which
this rule does not hold, but in most cases it will be
found to be a fair representation of the case.

A glance at the illustrations of the Chuka will show

History

how characteristic their physiognomy is, and a comparative vocabulary will also indicate Chuka as the meeting-ground of most of the peculiar phrases or words that can be traced definitely to Meru or Kikuyu.

CHAPTER II

HISTORY (*continued*)

THE foregoing theory of origins is offered with all diffidence, as a working hypothesis. It explains the existing conditions, and would seem to be borne out by the general evidence available. At the same time, there is no real proof that anything of the sort took place, and possibly some other explanation of existing facts will be found which contradicts the above.

Turning now to more certain ground, we come to the history of the country as given by native tradition. This is disappointing and scanty, owing to the fact that the natives, of all sections alike, seem to have made no sort of effort to preserve their history. Old men are to be found who remember a considerable amount of detail about the events of their youth, but only in a casual way, because they have some reason to do so. Sometimes they can include information about their fathers' times, but then it is generally owing to some claim in which they happen to be interested, which is based upon such events. Any sort of interest or pride in the previous history of their people seems to be almost entirely lacking. Songs, which might afford a source of information, become almost worthless

History

owing to the rapidity with which they change and are forgotten, and to the readiness with which one section will adopt the song of one of its neighbours. Genealogies, again, are depressingly difficult to obtain, and are vague and inaccurate in the extreme when obtained. Even when some old man is to be found who can give the names of four or five generations of his ancestors, it is seldom that he can give any detail at all about the people whose names he repeats, while he is more than likely to change one or two of the names about, on being asked again on some other occasion.

All this, of necessity, restricts the material available for anything like a consecutive history, for more than a very brief period of the past. Half-a-century is probably a fair estimate of the limit to native tradition ; beyond that, vague stories may be obtained, but the native inability to reckon time in the least accurately will very often lead to a story dating from ten years previously being related as an experience of the boyhood of the speaker's grandfather.

With a little care, however, it is possible to pick out certain elderly men who can give a fairly consecutive and coherent account of their early days, and from such men, using their information to corroborate previously obtained details, it is possible to secure a more or less definite and reliable history of early days.

From the vague mass of confused petty fights, raids, migrations and squabbles, the following main facts seem to stand out. They are agreed upon by informants from the various sections, who, happily, have no sort of false modesty about admitting the utter defeat of their kinsmen on some occasion, a fact which makes corroborative evidence much easier to obtain.

It seems certain that the Chuka were originally far more numerous and powerful than they are at present; they have undeniably been driven back from their old borders, and all the evidence goes to show that they have lost a considerable amount of territory. Various factors seem to have contributed to this result, the chief being apparently the growing pressure from outside, combined with unusual famine and disease among the Chuka.

The most important of the raids upon the Chuka was one which took place apparently somewhere about the middle of the nineteenth century; this came from the north, and was made by a combined force of Meru and Mwimbe. It seems to have originated in some quarrel which resulted in the expulsion of a fairly important man in Chuka. This man took refuge in Meru, where he remained for some little time, until he collected a numerous following of Meru and Mwimbe warriors, with whom he set out to re-establish himself in his old home. The expedition was entirely successful; taken, no doubt, largely by surprise, the Chuka were defeated and driven back over the Mara river, and across the Nithi; large quantities of stock and prisoners were taken, and the victors established themselves in the vacated country. The women who had been captured in the raid provided wives, and

History

others no doubt came from Meru or Mwimbe; the result was, that a separate section came into existence in the portion of country known as Muthambi; they call themselves Mwimbe, but admit relationship with the Chuka, with whom they are on friendly terms. They number about two thousand or so, all told, and have the same customs as the Mwimbe, slightly modified by Chuka influence.

This raid is the more interesting, as it is one of the rare examples of an expedition among these tribes having for its object the acquisition of territory rather than loot.

The second important raid upon the Chuka of which the details are to be obtained was an attack by the Embu. This took place about 1870, and was led by one Mtu wa Ikuru; and it was followed, in about 1890, by another raid, under a certain Njeru Karuku; the latter was a wizard living on the banks of the River Rupingazi, who appears to have combined the functions of wizard and war-leader in a very unusual way. These two attacks did not lead to any readjustment of boundaries, and were merely plundering expeditions. They, or at any rate the second one, resulted to some extent from irritation at the inroads of the Chuka, combined with a belief that the undertaking would be an easy one. During the last thirty years of the nineteenth century the Chuka appear to have suffered from a series of famines, together with an unusual amount of disease, both of human beings and of stock. This left them weak and also impoverished, and they tried to remedy the evil by small raids upon their neighbours. The latter retaliated, and found that their enemies were far feebler than they had supposed; hence the two attacks mentioned above.

The effect of this experience was to force the Chuka to take energetic means for their defence. They seem to have definitely decided upon a general scheme of action, embracing the whole country and entailing considerable labour. Curiously enough, no account can be obtained of any sort of general council or meeting at which the plan was adopted, nor is there any record of the name of the patriot who invented the method which served the Chuka in good stead at a time when they were in a precarious position.

The plan adopted consisted of a sort of general strengthening of the natural obstacles in the path of an enemy. The existing roads were destroyed or diverted to make them more defensible, while their steepest and most difficult points were strengthened by the erection of long tunnels of stakes and branches interwoven with growing trees; these led to small clearings, where the invader could be shot down with arrows as he emerged. The existence of the very steep and rocky gorges, which run the length of the Chuka country, served to make the roads thus defended almost impassable.

To the north-west, in the forest, a long line was created which should serve as a barrier to invaders who might wish to attack from that direction, coming, perhaps, from the Meru or Kikuyu country by the small paths in the forest. A long belt was formed of felled trees intermingled with growing ones, and further thickened with thorns and undergrowths; this was some forty or fifty yards wide, and must have been, when newly made, almost impassable to a raiding party not provided with serviceable axes. The remains of this barrier were still to be seen in 1912, about three or four miles above the edge of the forest.

Within these barriers the Chuka remained cut off from the intercourse with their neighbours which might have tended to destroy their peculiarities; they found that in their own country they were safe, but that as soon as they left it they were the prey of the other tribes. Similarly, they came to regard all travellers and strangers with suspicion, and they therefore became more and more exclusive and isolated. Such was their position when they first came into contact with European influence.

The first administrative post to be established in Kenya Province was Fort Hall, which was occupied in 1900. This controlled the Akikuyu proper, living to the west of the Tana, who had come into increased importance after the building of the railway. Constant friction going on between the Akikuyu on the west of the Tana and the Ndia Kikuyu living to the east, it was found necessary to undertake a small military expedition against these people; Chief Kutu was a prominent figure among them, and narrowly escaped with his life. This proved a lesson to him, and he has

History

since been a most useful friend to the Government, while his people appear to have quite accepted European control.

Shortly after this, the Embu took advantage of the peace in Chief Kutu's country to become much more daring and truculent in their attitude towards their neighbours. This necessitated the Embu Expedition in 1906, which effectually convinced the Embu of the futility of resistance, though no great loss of life resulted. Embu station was then established, first as a military station, and then as an administrative one. Subsequently it became obvious that the tribes still farther to the north would have to be brought under control, and Meru station was, therefore, established in 1908. The staff in each station being very small, authority over the various sections nominally in each district was at first very slight, and the outlying portions were hardly controlled at all for some little time; gradually, however, as the country and the people became better known, the authority of the Government became stronger. It was found, however, that the considerable distance between Embu and Meru left too large a section of natives without adequate control, and a sub-station was therefore established in Chuka in 1913. It will be seen from the foregoing details that the establishment of European authority is very recent, and that the whole administration of South-East Kenya is even yet in its infancy.

This position was not attained without some opposition on the part of the natives, though it is satisfactory to note that the stations at Meru and Chuka were established without military operations; on the whole, the bulk of the natives were glad enough, probably, to accept some settled form of government which would put an end to the perpetual raids and reprisals which went on in earlier times; and this attitude was no doubt more general owing to the absence of any definite fighting organization or caste, such as existed in South Africa. Still, the more daring and enterprising men resented the restriction on their movements, and even more, they resented the tax which they were expected to pay to maintain an authority which they disliked. This led to a considerable amount of passive resistance, which occasionally took the form of isolated attacks on Government servants; these, however, were never on a large scale, and seldom went beyond a few poisoned arrows shot from bushes. Still, the possibility of such attempts made prompt action necessary in such cases, and a few lives were lost in this way both among the natives and also Government servants.

The section which was probably most favourable to white control was the Emberre. Living in the plains of the Tana, they had no such natural defences as the other sections; while the very infertile and inhospitable nature of their country prohibited the existence of a dense population able to protect itself. Before European control had been established they were the victims of all their neighbours; the Masai, the Akikuyu, the Meru and the Akamba all attacked them at various times, while they were constantly at loggerheads with the Embu and Mwimbe. Still, they were not altogether defenceless, and on more than one occasion they were able to beat off attacks; indeed, they once succeeded (under the leadership of a remarkable woman, who seems to have acted the part of a local Joan of Arc) in beating off a raid by the Akamba, and following up the party across the Tana, where they recaptured the lost property, with additions.

The Eastern Embu and the Chuka remained for a long while very intractable, probably owing to the wooded and broken nature of the country; they never offered any real resistance, however, and rapidly yielded to the influence of money and trade as soon as their country began to be opened up.

The Lower Mwimbe also proved refractory, chiefly, no doubt, on account of the long distance between their country and any Government post until the opening of Chuka station.

The greatest amount of opposition, however, was from the Tharaka; isolated in their hills, at a considerable distance from any authority, they remained obstinately hostile and suspicious, for a considerable time. On several occasions they made unprovoked attacks on Government officials, but the opening up of the sections round them served to break down their prejudices; a determined official attitude soon persuaded them to accept the position of affairs.

So far, no white settlements have been formed on South-East Kenya, the land being far inferior to that on the north of the mountain, while the native population is also very dense.

The Church Missionary Society opened a station in Chief Kutu's country (Ndia Kikuyu) in 1910, and another a few miles to the north of Embu station in the same year; in neither case was the staff large, and the influence of these stations was therefore not very wide at first. These, with an Italian Roman Catholic Mission on the Mutonga river in Igoji, were the only European establishments existing on South-East Kenya, other than Government posts, at the outbreak of war; further missionary enterprise, however, has since taken place.

In addition to the methodical establishment of European influence as indicated above, there were also various occasions when white men travelled through the country; in each case the visit was a short one and had little effect upon the natives, though they do not seem to have had much reason for desiring a further acquaintance. Probably the first of these visits took place about the beginning of the last decade of the nineteenth century, or slightly earlier; no doubt careful investigation would enable the various parties to be identified, but there seems little to be gained thereby. The first time that the European was regarded as anything more than a passing phenomenon was when the railway was built, with the consequent foundation of the present town of Nairobi; this event seems to have been widely discussed, and the natives began to contemplate the European as a permanent factor in life; many, however, retained the idea that the white man was only a temporary visitor until quite recently; in fact, there are probably plenty of natives still, who expect him to disappear again as suddenly as he came.

Another alien influence of considerable importance was the Swahili explorer and slave raider from the coast; these people no doubt visited Kenya long before any white man had ever heard of the mountain; travelling up the valley of the Tana, a caravan would have found an excellent hunting-ground for slaves in Mwimbe and Emberre, before passing on to the Kikuyu country. Such expeditions were by no means always successful, and probably many of them left the coast only to be swallowed up by some unknown fate. Evil in object and effect though such enterprises were, it is impossible not to admire the courage and determination of these handfuls of ill-armed men who were travelling many hundreds of miles into the interior when the first European explorers were only just planning their inland expeditions.

The influence of such visitors was, however, probably slight; beyond a certain quantity of trade goods, a dislike of strangers and a considerable amount of disease, they seem to have left little to mark their presence, though the effect would vary with the locality, no doubt.

In addition to this intercourse, there was some little trade, at a very remote time, in beads, cowries and such things; these would be brought up from the coast

History

by tribes nearer the sea, and no doubt proved attractive novelties to the natives living on Mount Kenya, restricted as they were to iron ornaments almost exclusively. The old clumsy blue and white beads, of a type now seldom sold, are still common among all sections, chiefly as ornaments on the women's dresses.

To sum up, therefore, it may be said that the south-eastern slopes of Mount Kenya were very little affected by any alien influence until the beginning of the twentieth century.

Clans.—The social organisation of all the Embu tribes includes loose and vague grouping into families or clans. This arrangement, however, is not very conspicuous, and appears to have little actual effect except in the matter of marriage, union within the clan being regarded as incestuous. The clan is hereditary, the wife taking the husband's clan, as do the children. The members are supposed to be specially friendly and hospitable to each other. There appears to be a trace of what may be described as totemism : various animals and insects being regarded as the special signs of certain clans. This, however, does not appear to be of great importance, and it is quite common to find a man who knows his clan, but does not know of any special totem appropriate to it. In Ndia certain clans appear to have different hereditary characteristics. The Akiuru (totem, the frog) are regarded as being able to pronounce curses of special potency, though these can be guarded against by recourse to a doctor.

History

The Ithaga are the smiths, and appear to practise their art as an hereditary profession; they are also the masters of particularly potent curses, and in addition have influence over the rain, being able to detect its approach and to prevent it if they wish.

Certain other clans have special habits or restrictions; for instance, the Agachiku (totem, the ostrich) will not eat the breast of goats.

Among the Chuka fairly lengthy lists of clans can be obtained, but they are grouped in two sections, the Upper Chuka, living near the forest, being known as Thagana, and the Lower Chuka, living nearer the plains, being termed the Dumberi. These lists of clans may contain as many as thirty names, but it is unusual to find two men who will give the same list. I was not able to find any trace of totemism in Chuka, and the whole clan system seems to be obsolete and waning.

Somewhat akin to the clan system, but arising in a very different way, is the division of the men into ages. This, again, is vague and apparently unimportant. The Embu tribes certainly do not emphasize the system as do the main body of the Kikuyu, though I have on numerous occasions carefully collected lists of various ages according to their years. In Ndia there would seem to have been two ages to each year, but I never succeeded in getting any one list which tallied completely with any other. Each age is known by a particular name, which commemorates some characteristic of a period. In Emberre there is some trace of a rotation of names, a very old man sometimes giving the name

History

of his age as that of his grandson's age: the name was seemingly bestowed upon each group of initiates as they became warriors on circumcision. In Chuka it proved to be practically impossible to get any sort of list which was generally agreed upon.

This grouping into ages seems to have little practical result, and the association would appear to be sentimental rather than material. I have never been able to find any trace in Embu of the custom said to exist among the Kikuyu whereby the country is ceremonially handed over from an older to a younger age.

CHAPTER III

THE physical peculiarities of the Embu tribes, while not markedly different from those of their neighbours, nevertheless repay investigation. The various sections differ to some extent from one another, but the most marked characteristics will be found in the Chuka. Investigation seems to bear out the theory that the Chuka form the nucleus of primitive physical elements whose admixture with the Meru on the north-east, and the Kikuyu on the west, was responsible for the formation of the Embu tribes. The main characteristics which differentiate the Chuka from their neighbours in the matter of physique may be summed up as follows.

They are rather more thick-set and muscular than the other tribes, their weight being greater in proportion to their height. The size of the head is somewhat larger, although the cephalic index is nearly the same as that of their neighbours. Steatopygy is noticeable and the chest is well developed. The interocular distance is greater, and this latter detail gives a certain characteristic appearance to the Chuka face. Other peculiarities are : a greater amount of hair, a tendency to turn in the toes when walking, fingers and toes

Physical

thicker and shorter, and the big toe more separated from the others. Taking the Chuka as the section in which these peculiarities are most pronounced, the other tribes may be regarded as a kind of compromise between the Chuka and their numerous neighbours, the Meru on the north-east, the Kikuyu on the west and the Kamba to the south.

There is one very curious physical tendency to be found throughout the Embu tribes, but which is most marked among the Chuka, which is a tendency to irregularity of the fingers and toes. This may take the form of an extra toe or finger, while in other cases the fourth toe on each foot will be found noticeably shorter and less useful than the others. It is not uncommon to find this so marked that the owner in walking leaves a footprint showing only four toes.

The feature of the additional finger or toe is a very interesting one, which would repay full investigation. It occurs in all forms, from a nearly perfect finger, with nail, down to a mere lump of skin at the side of the hand or foot. The tendency is undoubtedly hereditary, and it is almost always found that several members of a family are equally affected. Oddly enough, however, the characteristic appears to be entirely confined to males. Although I must have seen many dozen cases of additional fingers I never saw it occur in a female. The natives, however, say that it has been known to occur in women, though very rarely. The tendency can, nevertheless, be transmitted through the female, and the man possessing it will often be found to have

Physical

a maternal grandfather or uncles similarly affected. The peculiarity is disliked by the natives, and where it takes the form of nothing more than a lump of skin, it is usually eliminated in early youth, by tying a piece of string tightly around the base, and this no doubt tends to obscure the frequency of its occurrence. I believe it to be correct to say that certainly one, and possibly two, per cent. of the Embu and Chuka are thus affected.

In appearance the Chuka, and to a somewhat less degree the Embu, may be described as decidedly darker in hue than their neighbours, the coloration of the eyes being the usual warm brown of the negro. There is, however, a curious light brown eye which is occasionally seen in Chuka. There are two characteristic casts of countenance: (1) which may be termed the bushman type, with projecting cheek-bones, lumpy forehead, heavy jaw and matted hair and beard, and (2) a sort of Mongolian type, with narrow eyes, high cheek-bones, wide mouth and a sloping forehead. These two types seem to be equally common, and are to be found even among different members of the same family.

I carried out a lengthy series of tests and measurements with a view to determining the degree of sensibility and perception of the senses. It is certain that these tribes, in common with the negro generally, have much less sensibility to pain than the ordinary European, this being due not to Spartan endurance, but to positive indifference. A man will walk about

Physical

with a dreadful festering sore on his leg or foot, and often will not take the trouble to visit a dispensary to get it dressed and bandaged, whereas the same sore in a European would mean great pain and confinement to bed. Again, the stoical indifference shown during the process of shaving with a piece of broken bottle, or still more during the ceremony of circumcision, cannot be attributed altogether to Spartan self-control; while there also seems to be a considerable measure of indifference to variations of temperature. Numerous tests with compass points on the finger-tips, the fore-arm and the shoulder-blades to determine the degree of ability to distinguish between pressure by one or two points, showed that the average native had per-ceptions little more than half as sensitive as the average European. Occasional instances of hypersensitiveness are to be met with, and I found one man who had a hypersensitive area all over his back from the neck to the knee, in which he could detect the difference between one and two points only two millimetres apart.

In colour-perception the native appears weaker than the European, though this is no doubt largely affected by inferior intelligence and training.[1] A number of pairs of coloured cards shuffled together would, as a rule, be fairly well sorted out in couples, though frequently slate and sepia or green and grey would be paired together, and where the subject was shown a card at one end of the room and was then told to fetch its mate from the other end of the room,

45

mistakes became very frequent. For general purposes, hearing and sight would seem to be about as accurate as those of Europeans, but not more so. Instances of short-sight or colour-blindness are extremely rare, while stammering is almost unknown. Perception among women is certainly less accurate than that of the men, while an odd feature is the extreme clumsiness of female fingers. Hardly any woman is able to pick up a small coin lying on a concrete floor; she has to get a pin or knife-point under the edge before her finger can grasp it. This is no doubt connected with the fact that the neatest handicrafts, notably the pretty bead-work, are practised by the men, although the women are capable of good and fine plaiting of mats and baskets.

The internal organs in the native appear to be wonderfully sound and efficient. Indigestion and dyspepsia seem to be unknown, and it is very rare to find any kind of kidney or bladder trouble. The lungs, however, appear to be vulnerable, bronchitis and pneumonia being frequent in occurrence and serious in results; were tuberculosis ever to gain a grip on these people it would, presumably, prove very fatal. The average native seems to be singularly wholesome blooded—that is to say, wounds and sores heal astonishingly well. A native will often recover comparatively rapidly from an accident which would certainly prove fatal to a European. Again, in the case of poisoned or gangrenous wounds, the most rudimentary attention in the way of dressings and antiseptics will produce

Physical

astonishingly rapid improvement. Syphilis and yaws are of distressingly frequent occurrence, there being presumably an hereditary infection of this kind; and this is, perhaps, responsible for the complications so frequently attendant upon childbirth; miscarriages are frequent, while the pains of labour are prolonged and acute. This fact, together with the great frequency of deaths in infancy, no doubt accounts for the smallness of the families. The average number of the adult children resulting from any marriage is probably little more than half the corresponding figure for European peasantry, and this astonishing fact is responsible for the very slow increase in population.

In muscular ability the Embu tribes are capable of far greater efforts than their somewhat unimpressive appearance would suggest. They are all good at jumping, though in this they are quite out-classed by the astonishing power of the Meru. As runners they are not particularly fast, but are capable of travelling enormous distances. On one occasion I sent a favourite runner with an urgent message to a brother official. My runner left at six o'clock at night and arrived back with the reply at ten o'clock the following night, completely exhausted, having covered ninety-two miles during that time, and this over native paths through fairly hilly country, and partly during the hours of darkness, with an appreciable risk from wild animals.[2]

The women are capable of astonishing weight-carrying feats. When fetching firewood or other

Physical

domestic loads they much prefer to carry a very large weight rather than make two journeys. On one occasion I found an old woman who had travelled eleven miles with a load of wood which when weighed proved to be one hundred and fifteen pounds. This was, of course, quite voluntary on her part, and she seemed highly amused when I told her that she would have been much wiser to have made two trips. It is obviously undesirable that these very heavy loads should be carried, and Government regulations rightly restrict the weight of a porter's load to forty-five pounds.

Physical development, on the whole, may be said to be fairly good, though it is in the form of wiriness rather than muscular development.

I carried out an exhaustive series of measurements and tests on the lines laid down by the British Association, and collected statistics of about one hundred and fifty men, and sixty boys; these were for the outstanding characteristics, such as height, weight, head and nose measurements, interocular distance, span, and the principal body measurements: also for colour-perception and other senses. I also measured, very fully, five adult males from each tribe, and took photographs to support these records. All these results were forwarded to the Royal Anthropological Institute (instruments used were by Hermann, of Zurich). An analysis of the features of greatest interest will be found in my article, " Some Notes on the Chuka Tribe," in *The Journal of the African Society* for 1916.

Physical

NOTES

[1] In these exercises I followed the general principles laid down by Doctoressa Montessori in her notes on the education of the senses.

[2] But Pheidippides is supposed to have travelled some 135 to 140 miles in the same time; though it is only fair.. to discount the stimulating effect of his interview with the God Pan (*Herodotus*, Book VI., Chapter 106).

CHAPTER IV

LAW

THE outstanding characteristic of the legal system of the Embu tribes is that which exists throughout a very large part of Africa—that is to say, the existence of civil law, almost to the exclusion of criminal law. The dominating idea in considering any offence is compensation for injury done. In the great majority of cases the infliction of punishment is scarcely considered, except in the shape of payment of a fine to repair the damage done. In this way a murderer is regarded as having inflicted a serious injury upon the relatives of his victim, and this he must repair as far as possible by a substantial payment in live stock. European legal procedure, in the shape of execution of the murderer without payment of compensation to the victim's relatives, appears to the native futile and pointless, since no effort is made to repair the damage done, while a useful man is destroyed for no purpose. This dominating idea of compensation, without deterrent punishment, is so firmly established in the native mind that it is most difficult to induce the native to see any sort of logic in the white man's procedure.

Law

By an extension of this compensation theory, the fine which was paid to the family of a murderer's victim was equally due from the family of the murderer should he himself be unable to meet it, or generally, fines due from an individual were due from the group to which he belonged. While this system probably worked satisfactorily enough when a native community was small and exclusive, it manifestly must lead to frequent injustice under more modern conditions, where the individual is no longer closely and permanently identified with his clan. For instance, I have known a case of a native returning home after ten months' work, hundreds of miles away at the coast, who found, on arrival at his village, that his satisfactory accumulation of wages was all swallowed up in payment for a crime committed by his brother some three months previously. It is, therefore, obvious that the rigid maintenance of the native system is impossible, though if any use is to be made of their existing social organization the change from the conception of compensation under civil law to deterrent punishment under criminal law must be cautious and gradual.

The courts which existed to administer native justice consisted of various Elders' Councils. These were not restricted to particular localities, but were formed as required from the qualified elders. Admission to this rank was obtainable only when a man had attained a certain age, which the father of two circumcised sons was regarded as having reached. Before admission a payment had to be made to the local elders, and a definite ceremony of admission was necessary, this being sometimes refused in the case of unsuitable men. Incapacity or poverty, therefore, occasionally excluded an old man otherwise qualified, and such people were termed *karanja*, the council of the elected elders being known as the *kiama*. In addition to the *kiama*, there was also a vague body of married men known as the *njama*, while the young warriors were also nominally grouped in matters concerning themselves. Of these, however, the recognized authority was the *kiama*, and these old men laid down the observations of the customs to be followed by the tribe in matters spiritual and temporal, though the other sections might be consulted in matters specially concerning them. The most potent weapon of the Elders' Council was their combined curse, which was regarded very seriously, since it was believed to have frequent fatal results. They also had the power of purging the minor cases of uncleanness, while their ranks frequently included one or more doctors.

It will be observed that this system places the social power in the hands of a group of old men, with the obvious disadvantage that it was unsuited to vigorous action in the shape of tribal defence or offence. To get over this difficulty there existed an individual known as a *muthamaki*, or war leader, generally a seasoned and experienced warrior. Upon this man or men depended the defence of the community and the organization of the raids which might be contemplated against a neighbouring tribe. These people tended to grow more important in troublous times, when a strong character and success in warfare might well give them such importance that they quite overshadowed the Elders' Council. In such cases, however, their rapid lapse into extortion and tyranny soon threw public sympathy and support back to the elders. The situation, in fact, would appear to have been something like that described in the Book of Judges, where authority alternated between the strong man, such as Samson, and the judge, such as Samuel, with recurrent periods when no authority was firmly established and " Every man did that which was right in his own eyes."

On the establishment of European administration, the local *athamaki*, or war leaders, were, in many cases, put forward as the spokesmen of their people, largely to the exclusion of the Elders' Council, with the result that the people were for some considerable time organized under native chiefs, and it was not until further experience was gained that the Elders' Councils were fully recognized, the head man being retained for convenience in administration; the old native system and modern European methods thus meeting in a separation of the judicial and administrative powers.

It will be noticed that the above organization contains no mention of the women. This is natural enough, since the general native view is that woman is always a minor and must be represented by some male legal guardian. Nevertheless, their opinions were by no means overlooked, the old women in

Law

particular having a considerable weight in the tribal councils. On one occasion, in Mwimbe, I became so exasperated with the incompetence and corruption of the local Elders' Council that I told them they were quite unfit to rule their people, and that unless they improved it would be necessary to consider whether the old women would not manage matters better. I was amused on my next visit to that area to be met by a party of old ladies, who had come to ask whether the local elders had improved or whether the change was really to be made. The threat had a salutary effect, being the cause of general merriment to such an extent that it spurred on the old men to a far higher level of efficiency.

I have already referred (p. 36) to a woman in Emberre, of the name of Churume, who, in a time of great danger and distress from Akamba raids, assumed the part of a local Joan of Arc, and headed a most successful raiding party into the enemy's territory, which resulted in the recovery of a considerable number of captives and stock, and established her firmly as the principal authority in her section. In 1910 this remarkable old woman of dominating personality was still alive, and as autocratic as ever, though then very old.

The working of native courts, such as they were, was somewhat peculiar. Since their awards almost always took the form of a payment by one party to the other, they must be regarded as courts of arbitration or upholders of moral standards rather than as authorities for the infliction of punishment. They had neither the will nor the means to imprison an offender, and only in the case of a notorious public nuisance or social outcast would they sanction the death penalty. Corporal punishment also was not inflicted. Their action, indeed, was really based more upon eventual Divine authority, though no very definite claim to this was made. Since, however, the tribal laws were universally supposed to have emanated originally from the Creator, it was considered that an award pronounced by an Elders' Council was tantamount to an interpretation of the Divine law, so that non-compliance with it rendered the offender liable to all the misfortunes which threatened the transgressor of tradition. In itself such a view may be considered as a fine and austere conception : unfortunately in actual practice the elders who interpreted the system were very seldom equal to upholding its dignity.

The native conception of admissible evidence is also curious and disconcerting. The story told to a witness by his father or grandfather, possibly years previously, is regarded as excellent evidence, while it is also very hard to differentiate between the actual facts as they occurred and the native witness's idea of the facts as they should be. For instance, a plaintiff may claim the return of three goats given by his father to the defendant. The transaction having taken place some years previously, these three goats will probably have increased to, say, fifteen. The plaintiff, therefore, not only claims fifteen goats, but talks as though his father

Law

had originally paid fifteen goats. The defendant, on the other hand, knows that he took the goats only temporarily for herding, and that they were shortly afterwards unfortunately killed by a leopard. He therefore maintains that he never received the goats at all. This tendency to take short cuts in evidence produces a most confusing effect. In such cases both speakers will honestly consider that their statements are the absolute truth, flatly contradictory though they may be to the mind of the European listener. Only the most patient investigation will enable one to arrive at the true facts, and it may well be urged, therefore, that the general belief in the native's essential untruthfulness is unfair. He will certainly frequently lie with fluency and audacity, but in an actual court case before his own Elders' Council, it is my experience that he will generally speak what he considers to be the truth to the best of his ability, largely distorted though his conception of it may be.

No account of the Embu legal organization can omit one important factor, the wizard. At first sight it may not be obvious how this sinister figure is concerned with the law or tradition, but it must be remembered that all law is theoretically based on Divine instructions, and that such penalties as exist are of a supernatural or spiritual form. The Elders' Council enforces its decrees by means of a curse, and thus it has a close relation to the performances of a wizard, who also claims to have Divine instruction as the basis of his art. (The position and functions of the wizard will be

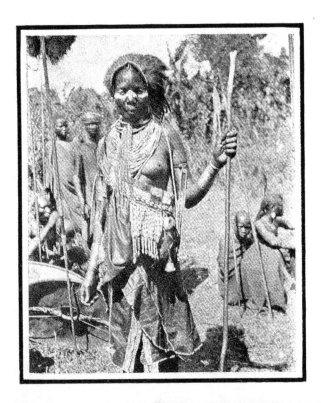

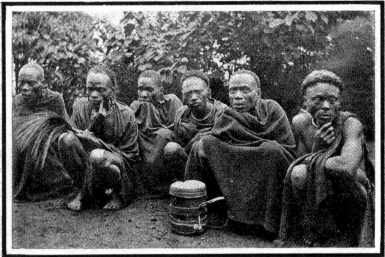

FEMALE OPERATOR FOR GIRLS' INITIATION, MWIMBE.

Note the ceremonial chalk marks round the eyes, to prevent the glance bringing misfortune.

SOME MEMBERS OF A CHUKA KIAMA (ELDERS COUNCIL).

Towards the left is seated the leader with his badge of office, a whisk made of a tail. In front is a small bottle of honey—a present for the writer.

Law

found more fully discussed in the chapter "Magic.") It is certainly the case that the Elders' Councils were very often influenced, if not dominated, by an important "Doctor," and the fact that any elder was reputed to be able to perform the necessary purification for the milder forms of ceremonial uncleanness, probably tended to make the old men sympathetic towards a wider use of magic or mystical powers.

Descriptive : A Court Case.—The following case is given at length, since it may be of interest as showing the working of the native mind. As far as possible, it is kept in exactly the form in which it occurred, and may be regarded as a typical example of the sort of case which arises almost every day.

It is one which is being heard before the Council of Elders, locally known as the *Kiama*. As already explained, this body is the native court which was in old days supposed to settle all matters in dispute; under white administration an attempt is made to utilize the services of these old men to deal with all cases of a trifling nature, or in which details of native custom are of importance.

We will suppose that, in the present case, the *kiama* concerned (there is a *kiama* for each section) has been unable to settle the point in dispute; but since the case is one governed entirely by native custom, they have been called in to the station to sit and hear the matter again, in an endeavour to arrive at some settlement.

On a level patch of grass, in the shade of a con-

57

Law

venient tree, sit the thirty old men who are concerned
in this particular matter. They may number more, or
in simple cases quite a small bench is considered
sufficient; it is largely a matter for individual settlement, according to the details of each action. The
plaintiff and the defendant are both strongly represented by the elders from their own particular part,
some of whom are probably their own relatives; as
many as possible of these are got in, since they have
an indirect interest in the matter, and therefore are
all the more likely to be favourable. Close to them,
though not of their own circle, are the two parties
to the suit, while various friends and assistants attend
in case of need. Witnesses are also present, though
the local idea of evidence is so peculiar that very little
of what is said would be considered relevant in an
English court.

Court fees, in the shape of a goat to be eaten by the
elders, have already been paid by both parties, for the
first hearing; but since the second hearing has become
necessary, the fees have to be paid over again, since
"the elders have become hungry again," one of the
mottoes of the court being: "An empty stomach has
no ears."

These important preliminaries having been satisfactorily settled, the elders dispose themselves for the
interminable sitting which is always considered necessary. They form themselves into a ring, in the centre
of which the speaker of the moment stands—or rather
dances, for frantic gesticulation and dramatic posturing

Law

are most necessary for impressive oratory. Snuff is consumed by the circle in large quantities, and if they are Chuka, a pipe circulates from time to time. Those members who are not specially interested, fall placidly asleep, to be aroused at the more important points by the inevitable clamour from all present. As a rule, the principal part is taken by a few of the more energetic or more interested elders, while " the rude forefathers of the hamlet sleep " until it is necessary to take some active part in the proceedings.

This state of affairs is presumably responsible for the constant calls for attention, and pauses for a response, which interrupt every speech. A relation of facts —or alleged facts — becomes a series of questions, of which the answers are repeated after the speaker. This makes the conduct of the trial intolerably slow, since the essential portions of any speech are simply lost in the surrounding verbal trimmings. The proceedings are opened by an elder, who springs to his feet and takes the centre of the circle; he walks round and round, talking as loudly as he can, his voice at the more important points rising to a screech, while the argument is emphasized by waving arms and thumps on the ground with the stick which he carries. To translate literally :

" I say, ye elders, do you hear me ? I ask, do you hear me ? "

(*Muttered reply :*) " We hear you."

" I tell you, this man—this man here, do you see ? " (*Pointing to the plaintiff.*)

59

Law

(*Reply:*) " We see."

" This man here had a goat. Some goats. How many goats? " (*Holding out a hand with the fingers arranged to show the number of goats.*)

(*Reply by such old men as take the trouble to look:*) " Three."

(*Orator, triumphantly:*) " Yes, three; three goats; three."

And so on, throughout the speech, while the old man stumps excitedly round the circle, waving his arms, thumping the ground, and shrieking out his points in a cracked falsetto.

In this tedious fashion the details of the claim are given. It seems that the plaintiff lent two goats to the defendant three years ago; or rather, the goats were left as security for a debt in which a spear and a pot of honey figure vaguely. The debt was duly redeemed, but the defendant refused to give back the two goats, together with one kid that had been born in the interval. (A long explanation at this point is necessary, to account for one he-goat and two kids, that died.) The plaintiff, therefore, claims the three goats.

The defence now begins. Firstly, the goats were never left as security, but they were to be pastured by the defendant, who, in return for his trouble, was to have all the increase during the time that the goats were left with him. The debt was quite a separate affair, and, in any case, it had never been settled, since only the spear had been given back, and that a very poor one; the pot of honey was still due. At this point an

Law

interminable wrangle ensues as to the number of births and deaths that took place in the goat family during the three years.

Some eight hours having been spent very pleasantly in this way, the elders decide that they are unable to give judgment for either party; they therefore require a trial by ordeal, which will take the form of licking a red-hot knife to see whose tongue blisters the most. A neighbouring " wise man " is got in to make the preparations, and both parties solemnly lick the hot iron, after which they parade round the circle with their tongues stuck out for all to see and judge of the burns. It is unanimously agreed that the defendant's tongue is far more blistered than that of the plaintiff, so the three goats are duly awarded to the latter. The decision is generally regarded as being very satisfactory and incontrovertible, even the defendant acquiescing, though reluctantly.

To European ideas the whole affair is simply ludicrous: but it must be remembered that in this particular case it was probably utterly impossible to come to any decision by logical methods, and the ordeal at any rate presents a means of settlement which is uncomplainingly accepted by both parties, neither of whom would have been in the least content if he had been told that the case was " Dismissed for lack of Evidence," by a white judge. Naturally, such methods cannot be allowed in serious cases, but for the settlement of minor disputes the old-established native custom has many advantages.[1]

Law

[1] " Their domestic affairs—marriages, adoptions, inheritances and so forth—continued to be regulated by their own spiritual guides, in accordance with their own sacred books, and were seldom, if ever, brought before a Muhammadan Kazi.   On the other hand, the conquerors naturally kept in their own hands the administration of the criminal law. . . ."   (The Mogul policy towards their Hindu subjects, as described by Sir R. K. Wilson in his *Digest of Anglo-Muhammadan Law.*)

CHAPTER V

LAND TENURE

THE system of land tenure around Embu is a curious and somewhat anomalous one, particularly puzzling on first acquaintance. The Bantu tribes of Africa, as a whole, of course, are inclined towards a more or less communal land system, and private ownership of land is, therefore, as a rule, practically non-existent in the form in which it is understood in Europe. In the case of the tribes about Mount Kenya, however, the usual Bantu system is considerably modified.

After much investigation and consideration I am inclined to believe that the explanation of the existing system lies in the history of the settlement of the area by the tribes now inhabiting it. There can be little doubt that these tribes are all descended from immigrants who arrived at no remote date. The peaceable outlook of the new-comers induced them to effect occupation by agreement with the original inhabitants rather than by conquest and slaughter. There is a definite and widespread tradition of the existence of the original inhabitants, the Agumba, who were forest-dwelling, hunting people. On the arrival of the pastoral and agricultural immigrants the land was

63

Land Tenure

taken over from the Agumba by what was practically a system of purchase. The forest was gradually felled, more and more being brought into cultivation, until we reach the existing state of affairs when the Agumba have disappeared, and the land is held by the descendants of the original immigrants.

This system of purchase is no doubt responsible for the very large measure of individual possession which exists in the present system of land tenure. The original new-comer, who bought a considerable tract from its hunting owners for some more or less nominal payment, handed down the tradition of this purchase to his descendants, who, therefore, regard themselves as having a definite and individual right to the piece of land in question, and in this way practically every piece of land has a theoretical individual owner.

This arrangement, however, is certainly alien to the general principle of more or less communistic tenure which characterizes the Bantu, with the result that the two opposing systems produce considerable uncertainty and conflict, to an extent which probably renders a clear comprehension of the land system difficult for even the wisest and most experienced native. This I believe to be the explanation of the puzzling nature of the whole question, and the frequent anomalies with which the inquirer meets.

The question of land tenure is, to some extent, bound up with that of the position of women in native society, and also the general laws of inheritance. Both these kindred subjects must be taken into consideration when dealing with land.

The general principle may be described as individual ownership in a fairly definite form, rather than either communism or feudalism, though this individualism in practice is largely modified by the constant action of the weight of general tradition, which tends to break down actual personal ownership.

It will be found in practice that any piece of land is, as a rule, the subject of three separate claims. Firstly, the real ownership; secondly, the claim of the tenant; thirdly, the claim of the woman who has cultivated it. In this connection the land falls into one of two categories—cultivated or uncultivated. In practice, however, this division only affects the third claim— the temporary one of the relation of the woman to the product of her labour.

The original owner may be in theory quite an important landlord, with a claim to a large area, and it is not unusual to find comparatively insignificant people who are supposed to own large tracts of country. This right, however, is held cheaply, and may be satisfied by an almost nominal payment; thus the ground landlord is often content with the single payment of a large pot of beer for the right to occupy several acres. Once this is paid, the tenant has the right to cultivate or build upon the land, and the ground landlord would probably find it in practice very difficult to expel him as long as the land was usefully employed. This would seem in fact to be due to the weight of general Bantu law—

E   65

Land Tenure

that the land should be held for the good of the community—tending to modify the local principle of individual ownership. The working tenant having thus acquired his land, it becomes necessary to clear it and bring it under cultivation. The heavy work of this, such as the felling of trees, the destruction of bush and the eradication of roots and stones, falls to the man, but once cleared and fit for cultivation it is the woman who begins to have an interest in it. The husband must clear and prepare the land, but it is the wife who sows and reaps the crop. She thus obtains a very definite right to the produce of the field, and this is generally recognized, though naturally the right is a short-lived one, depending upon the crop. Nevertheless, the woman's interest in any field is fully admitted, and she carries it with her in case of marriage or removal to another home.

The general laws of inheritance would seem to apply very largely to land as well as to other property. Generally speaking, on the death of a man it is his brother that is his heir. This seems to be based upon the underlying principle that there are probably children whose rights require safeguarding, for whom the father's brother makes the best guardian. In the case of a brother inheriting, there seems to be reason for saying that he acquires a life-interest only. On his death the land reverts to the son of the original tenant, who also automatically becomes the guardian of his late father's wives, who have, of course, their own cultivation rights. As the son probably also has wives of his own, again with their cultivation rights, it is obvious that one man, with the women of his household, may well have definite interests in quite a number of different fields. This is the kind of situation which tends to make specific cases of land tenure so elusive and incomprehensible. In practice, the Elders' Council seem to settle any case brought before them on its particular merits in accordance with general principles; it is very difficult to induce them to lay down definite abstract rules. It will be seen, therefore, that in questions of purchase or compensation for land, there are two interests to be satisfied, first, that of the original owner, and second, that of the occupier, which carries with it the cultivation rights of the women concerned, and, if injustice is not to be done, these claims should all be considered. Thus, when I was engaged upon the construction of the Government Station in Chuka I paid some small compensation to fourteen occupants of the land required. The ground landlord, however, waived his claim since he was the nominal owner of a number of square miles; as he was profiting in other ways by the establishment of the station, he was prepared to forgo the pot of beer which technically, no doubt, should have been paid to him.

It must be remembered that it is difficult for the native to conceive of absolute and perpetual occupation of a piece of land. His wasteful method of cultivation necessitates letting his plantation revert to bush after it has been worked for a very few years, while the flimsy nature of his hut precludes any conception of

Land Tenure

permanent buildings. He can, therefore, hardly contemplate such complete and permanent loss of land as is entailed by the erection upon it of, say, a railway station or a church ; and it is this outlook which makes the native fatally ready to dispose of what a European regards as permanent land rights. In this way a native community will willingly and gladly part with a very large portion of their land, only to realize some years later that they have become extremely cramped for space. A feeling of resentment then springs up against the white men who have permanently occupied the old tribal lands, even though the natives themselves were willing and eager to make the original arrangement. From this arises the necessity for a close watch and control by Government over the alienation of native land, even against the immediate desires of the natives themselves.

Land is frequently the subject of charms, either to secure the fertility of the plantation or to ward off pests or marauders. It is very common to see the top of an earthen pot buried in the ground on the road bordering a field, or a bunch of leaves, grass, twigs, etc., may be hung up in a neighbouring tree, while a very common method of deterring intruders in Embu and Chuka is the erection of strings of creepers on poles, somewhat like a telegraph wire along the borders of the field. Passing uninvited under these lines is supposed to entail an attack of venereal disease on the intruder.

Timber, grazing and watering rights appear to be held in common, and the permission for access to a highly esteemed salt-lick for cattle has often been the cause of much quarrelling and discussion between two neighbouring tribes.

Under conditions of European civilization, the old native system of land tenure must, no doubt, be to some extent modified: the complicated details and trivialities of its old form will tend to disappear, while the outstanding principles will grow more definite. In the main, however, the system would seem well suited to native needs, and there appears to be no reason why it should not continue to control the administration of land in native possession: the principle that effective useful occupation alone justifies private ownership is well understood by the native, and it works on the whole very beneficially; it might, indeed, find advocates beyond the confines of Africa!

CHAPTER VI

THE general moral standard cannot be considered a high one: nevertheless, it is very definite, and works on the whole decidedly for the benefit of the community. Generally speaking, it may be described as the natural and wholesome standard; while sexual relationship is regulated only by easy-going laws, the strongest opposition is shown to anything out of the normal course of nature, such as connection with immature children or unnatural vices. Free love is by no means permitted, though there is no objection to extreme intimacy short of actual sexual connection, to which fact is probably due the very general idea that complete freedom exists. Under native customs severe penalties were inflicted upon offenders against the general moral standard, the Chuka being the most particular in this respect. A child resulting from the union of an uninitiated boy and girl was destroyed, while the parents were killed by having a stake thrust through them. Illicit union with an adult girl or married woman formed the ground of civil action by the injured party, either father or husband, and could be compensated by payment in stock. In the case of a warrior who seduced a girl the consequent

70

payment was taken into account in the consideration of the dowry, if he subsequently married her. While the moral standard is undoubtedly lax, there seems to be good ground for believing it to have been formerly less so; old men can freely be heard regretting the increasing laxity.

On the whole, the women may be described as usually faithful to their husbands. Genuine affection between husband and wife is by no means uncommon, while an attractive characteristic is the real love between parents and children. Prostitution under tribal conditions is unknown, although, with the advance of civilization, there is an increasing tendency for women to go to the towns as prostitutes or to live in concubinage with strangers.

Marriage between relations was strictly prohibited to a far wider degree than is the case among Europeans. Members of the same clan were even prohibited from marriage, although no actual relationship of any degree could be traced. Blood brotherhood or adoption had the same effect as actual relationship.

Rape was regarded as a serious offence, and was uncommon: the offence could be expiated by a payment to the relations, though, here again, subsequent marriage discussions would take this into account. The circumstances would be considered by the Elders' Council in making their award, which would probably be a fairly heavy fine on the offender.

Polygamy is fully authorized by custom, but is carried out in practice only to a limited degree, largely owing, no doubt, to the expense of the numerous dowry payments. In very many cases men may be found to have only one wife, though three or four are not uncommon, while a wealthy man may have twenty or thirty. This is by no means unpopular with the women themselves, as it adds importance to the common establishment and lightens the general work. An old man with several young wives will also generally take a lenient view on the subject of their faithfulness. The first wife is styled the Big Wife, and she retains a certain seniority and importance in the household. She is by no means averse from her husband taking additional wives, and I have frequently known such women to urge their elderly husbands to marry an additional young wife so that she may help with the housework. The senior wife is not supposed to marry again in the case of the death of her husband, and this explains the general native repugnance to the remarriage of the Christianized native widow.

Divorce is a matter of arrangement, and it is difficult to specify any definite grounds for it. Unfaithfulness is certainly one, but much more general reasons were frequently accepted which could only be described as incompatibility of temper. In the case of a divorce the husband was entitled to the return of the actual animals paid as dowry, and in former times it was considered disgraceful for a parent to sell the stock obtained as his daughter's dowry, since these animals represented a definite bond between the woman and her parental village. Divorces, on the whole, are uncommon, and tribal law certainly intended marriage to be a permanent union. It is much to be regretted that there is a strong modern tendency to break down the former strictness. While it is no doubt desirable to raise the status of women, it is very startling to the native mind to find that, while he regards woman as a perpetual minor, under the guardianship and supervision of a male relative, European law, on the contrary, regards her as having the same rights, privileges and freedom as a man, and this revolutionary change naturally has a great tendency to encourage the women to throw off the restraint, with most unfortunate consequences. The alteration in the status of women must therefore be carried out cautiously and gradually if the whole moral standard of the native is not to be broken down. Only too often Europeans who honestly believe themselves to be encouraging native women to assume greater responsibility and self-expression are merely inducing the unfortunate creatures to assume a position and a mode of life which must result in degradation and misfortune.

In all disputes connected with marriage, or offences relating to such matters, the question is settled by a payment in live stock; it may, therefore, be wondered that I do not add a Table showing the penalty for each offence, as has been to some extent done for the larger and more important tribes. I have not done so, as it appears to me to be merely misleading in the case of the minor tribes: mostly poverty-stricken and handicapped in cattle-breeding, they cannot be expected to possess laws which entail penalties far beyond the wealth of any but the richest members of the community. In practice, I believe the fines to have been largely modified according to the power of the loser to pay; certainly I was never able to obtain any definite scale of numbers, though occasionally informants would give a rough number for an imaginary case.

Dowry.—The system of payment, usually in live stock, for a wife, obtains throughout the Embu tribes just as it does through so much of Africa. This dowry system is sometimes alluded to as the purchase of a wife, but this description is misleading and unfair, for it represents the woman in the light of a slave or chattel, which is far from being the case. Were the dowry payment an actual purchase price, the wife could obviously be subsequently sold again by her husband, which is certainly not the case. The reason of the dowry payment would appear to be a species of guarantee. On the one side, it ensures fair treatment by the husband, who might otherwise be called upon to set free his wife with the loss of the dowry in addition, while on the other side, it tends to ensure good behaviour on the part of the woman, since her relations are all interested in her faithfulness, lack of which might entail upon them the return of the dowry to the aggrieved husband. It must also not be forgotten that the woman herself has considerable freedom of choice in her husband. I have frequently known of cases where a woman flatly refused to accept an advantageous match urged by her relations.

Marriage Laws

On the whole, the system must be said to work well, and where, through poverty or stock disease, the dowry system has broken down it will generally, I believe, be found that the standard of morality and marital fidelity has suffered correspondingly.[1]

The amount paid as a dowry varies very largely according to the wealth of all concerned. In addition to this, there are certain somewhat obscure complications in the payments which add very much to the difficulty of laying down any definite rules. Chief amongst these is what may be termed the fertility payment, in which an initial sum on marriage is subsequently supplemented by further payments on the birth of children, while it is possible to find this arrangement continued even to grandchildren. In such cases payment is obviously long delayed, with the inevitable result of subsequent disagreements and lawsuits. In a word, dowry payments may be said to provide the greater part of the civil legal work of the community. Nevertheless, the breakdown of the system would be a real disaster, at any rate until it has been replaced by some other arrangement equally acceptable to the native mind; and of this there are at present no signs. For this reason the marriages of converts under European law frequently turn out most unsatisfactory. Since it is unlikely that all the bride's relations are also converts, a portion at any rate of her family regard her marriage as void; this inevitably weakens the regard of the woman herself for the sanctity of the tie, with the result that the formal marriage before the Magistrate

75

comes to be regarded as less binding than one carried out according to tribal custom, although the reverse might have been expected.

Generally speaking, the women will be found most tenacious of their rights. Although they have in a way an inferior and subordinate position, they nevertheless realize most fully what they are entitled to, and will show themselves more tenacious in holding to their rights than will the men of the tribe. The influence of the women of the tribe is also strongly conservative. They cling to the old native dress far more than the men do, and they are also very ready to raise objections to the introduction of novelties which concern their work—for instance, the use of European-made iron hoes in cultivation. Innovations in matters mainly concerning the men will be, as a rule, readily accepted : the use of matches has very rapidly displaced the old fire-stick; but where the women are concerned, novelties, such as improved agricultural methods, will generally be stoutly resisted.

The dowry system is very firmly rooted in the native mind, and it may be said to work, on the whole, for the benefit of all concerned; any innovation or change of system would have to be introduced with great caution, if the risk of serious harm to native morals is to be avoided. This point is well worth attention from missionaries and educationalists, who are sometimes liable to overlook the useful aspect of the dowry system; with the result that Christian marriages are very apt to be regarded by the heathen relatives as irregular and negligible, a view which is bound to have some effect upon the couple themselves. There would seem to be no very strong argument against the dowry in the case of all marriages, and those who urge its abolition should realize that, in native eyes, they are practically recommending concubinage. The Elders' Councils understand the system perfectly, and there seems no reason why it should not endure, with certain modifications.[1]

NOTE

[1] For a striking example of this see the author's article, "The Tsetse Fly and Native Morals," in *The Journal of the African Society* for October 1923.

CHAPTER VII

Birth

THE first part of a native's life may be said to consist of the years from birth up to initiation. During this time the child is a minor, and is not considered as a member of the community, but is relegated to an inferior position and largely absolved from responsibility. It remains more or less under the control of the women, and may not eat with adults. The circumstances attending the birth are of considerable importance, and certain accidents connected therewith are "unlucky"—the child should not touch the ground at delivery, for instance—while any peculiarity at birth is to be deplored. In particular, the presence of teeth in a new-born child is regarded as most unfortunate, while great importance is also attached to the cutting of the lower or upper teeth first; indeed, irregularity in this matter was formerly liable to lead to the destruction of the unfortunate infant. Twins were also regarded with great disfavour (they occur but rarely, however), and one or both might be condemned to death by exposure.

Considerable importance is thus attached to the actual birth, and various ceremonies have to be observed;

78

the women of the village take a keen interest in the event, and it is by no means the casual occurrence that it appears to be in some other parts of the world.

The child's name is fairly definitely regulated by custom, and is generally hereditary according to certain rules. These differ slightly among the sections, but roughly, the following is the system. For a son, the eldest is called after the father's father; the second, after the mother's father; the third and successive sons are called after the parents' uncles and brothers. For a daughter, the eldest is called after the father's mother; the second, after the mother's mother; and the remainder are called after aunts.

Sometimes, however, a name may prove unlucky— *i.e.* the child dies. In this case, a doctor is sometimes consulted, and he frequently advises that the next child should be called, not by the name which it should have, according to system, but by the name of an animal. In this case, certain sections regard the child as having some occult connection with its name animal, and, in consequence, both the child and the father are forbidden to harm the animal in any way; this, however, seems to be an old and obsolete belief, as many natives will deny that there is any restriction on killing the animal concerned. A name is sometimes altered by the women when the child begins to show its character, but this would seem to be little more than a nickname.

On circumcision, a boy receives a new name, as an adult, by which he should subsequently be known; though in practice the former one generally persists

Periods of Life

in conversation. The new name is derived from the
" godfather " who supports the boy during the operation of circumcision, and it usually denotes some
peculiarity or incident connected with the old man's
life. The prefix *mundu a* (man of . . .) is always
used, so that the boy may start life as Njeru, and, on
circumcision become " Mundu a Thara," although
he may continue to be colloquially known as " Njeru."
The father's adult name is added, if it is necessary, to
distinguish the person meant; so that one may have
some such handy name as Mundu a Igichania wa
Mundu a Mutua, as a certain elder in Chuka was
called.

The observances attending a birth differ somewhat
among the various sections; the following account of
the customs in Mwimbe may be taken as a type, though
it is rather more elaborate than the others.

When a woman is about to give birth her friends
come in and await the event. When the child is born
one of the women cuts the umbilical cord, wraps the
child in grass, and places it by the side of the hut wall
outside. Afterwards they return and utter trills, four
for a girl and five for a boy. All the women then, on a
prearranged plan, call out : " This is Nyagga," or : This
is the daughter of So-and-so." After this the mother
and child stop four days in the hut. On the fourth day
any hair on the child is shaved, and if the child is a girl
she is taken outside and given a small piece of stick,
which is then broken into pieces, and the pieces are
placed close to the fireplace. In the case of a boy, he is

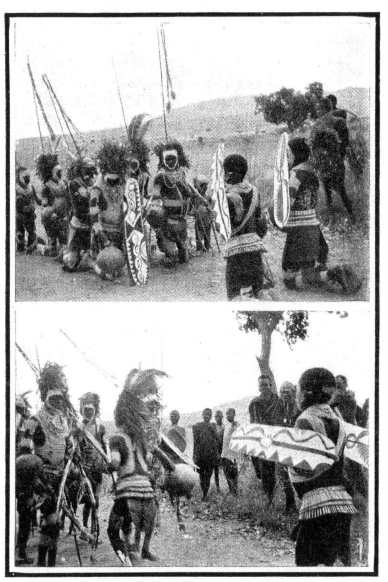

EMBERRE BOYS' PRE-INITIATION DANCE.

1.—Note the black charcoal patches round the eyes to prevent the glance having any
evil effect; and the white clalk ring round the faces to prevent the words having the
force of a curse.

2.—Note the elaborate chalk and clay painting of the body; also the feather
headdresses and reed waist fringes.

given a miniature bow and arrows, which are also afterwards placed close to the fireplace. After that the father goes to the plantation and digs yams, and the mother makes porridge: the father leaves the yams on the plantation. The next morning the mother and child go with a gourd to the plantation and take the yams and put them into a basket; the mother then pretends to feed the child on the porridge and takes the yams home. A few days later she makes a feast in the evening. First the child is shaved and the hair is put away in the hut; then a party of children come and are given bananas and yams: grass is taken from the thatch over the door and the bananas and yams are cooked. The child's hair is then burned in the fireplace, and the ashes are trampled on by the children, who say: " To-day we eat the hair of the child of one of us." This completes the ceremony.

When the teeth begin to appear a half-gourd is taken and a goat is pierced in the neck with a small arrow. The resultant blood is caught in a pot, and in another pot some honey is put. The mother then makes a large quantity of porridge and all her women friends come to eat it. The mother dips the second finger of the right hand into the blood and smears it four times on the child's teeth, subsequently doing the same thing with the honey, which is also rubbed from the tip of the nose over the head to the nape of the neck. Four days later, four cowrie shells are taken and put round the child's neck, with two strings of beads. The blood left in the gourd is mixed with flour by the mother and

Periods of Life

one old woman, the mixture being then cooked and eaten by these two, which completes the necessary ceremonies for the child.

In the above account it will be noticed that the numbers " four " and " five " recur : these numbers are the same in the ceremonies for all sections, and also occur in some other connections. I am unable to offer any explanation of them; the natives, when asked, only say that the custom was dictated by their forefathers.

In addition to the ritual attending the actual birth, there is also the obscure ceremony known as " Goat Birth " among the Kikuyu; or among the minor tribes *Kuitwa Ya Nyamu* (to be named of a beast). The details of this appear to vary considerably, and the rules governing it seem elastic. Broadly, it takes place in early infancy, though the Chuka seem inclined to postpone it somewhat.

A doctor is summoned and the mother sits on the floor of the hut, while a goat is killed. The skin of this is then spread over the mother's legs, and the child is seated on it, facing the mother, after which the skin is wrapped round the child. A number of old women are present, and they then snatch the child from the skin, giving the trilling cry for a birth—five for a boy and four for a girl—and at the same moment the doctor may utter a name for the child. It seems obscure how far this is a new name, or whether it is usually given when the naming has been postponed. The goat's flesh subsequently provides a feast.

Periods of Life

There is a curious detail sometimes added: the intestine of the goat is tied round the mother's waist, and is cut at the moment when the child is taken up. From the skin of this goat is cut a sort of amulet for the child to wear, consisting of a strip from the fore and hind leg, while a diamond-shaped piece of skin is also left on the breast of the goat. The long strip is worn by the child over the shoulder, four days for a girl and five for a boy; it is then taken off and burned, the mother and child being shaved. The use of the diamond-shaped piece of skin from the breast is obscure: a similar piece, however, figures in other ceremonies, and serves to make a finger-ring.

The whole proceeding is curious and puzzling; the complete lack of any explanation, with the variation in detail among the sections, suggests that the ceremony is the remnant of some older and more elaborate ritual, which has now been almost lost: it is guarded with considerable jealousy, and the above account is from various informants, as I was never able to witness the proceedings myself.

The use of the *Rukwara* strap occurs on other occasions, and it would seem to be a general amulet or mascot.

Adolescence

When the child is nearly full grown, the time arrives for his or her definite recognition as an adult, and this takes the form of a species of circumcision.

The operation of circumcision for the boys, and the

equivalent ceremony for the girls, represents the initiation of the neophyte into the full body of the tribe. It is a ceremony of the first importance in the life of the child, while it also represents a great occasion for the parents. Very much is bound up with it, and a full comprehension of its position in the native system is necessary for any sympathetic understanding of native life. The line between the initiated and the uninitiated is of such moment that it is only natural that the performance of the ceremony should assume great importance both to the young people and to their parents.

Before the operation a ceremony takes place known as the *Mburre ya migumu*—the goat of the Migumu (wild fig) tree. The details of this vary to some extent: the following account is of the Chuka practice, which is fairly typical.

On the day before the circumcision, the father kills a goat, and from the skin he makes two straps, one from the hind leg, from hoof to belly, and the other from the other hind leg, from hoof to centre of back. These are worn by the boy or girl, round the neck, one hanging down in front and the other hanging down behind. This is done at the threshold of the house. Then the boy goes with all the other candidates, carrying nothing, to the forest to get leaves of the Migumu-tree. This is done by a friend who has not yet been through the ceremony, who climbs the tree and gets the leaves for all. This boy is given a present, usually some small ornament. The boys take a bunch of the leaves in each hand, and these must not be put down again. They are not tied in any way. The boys then return home, and each one seats himself in front of his father, who smears his face with chalk. The warriors then fetch him, and he goes to his mother's house and deposits the leaves on the roof, while he goes to eat. He then returns to fetch them, and he retains them until the next day, when he is operated upon, and the leaves are thrown away. A similar rite is gone through by the girls.

Before the actual ceremony is carried out, the candidates are carefully prepared for a considerable time beforehand by a selected elder. The boys carry out the dances appropriate in their situation and form a separate little community under the guidance and control of their old instructor. The teachings given at this period are somewhat vague, but may be described as consisting of the rules of the tribal morality and good behaviour. The young people are taught how to conduct themselves toward their elders and their relations generally, the complicated rules of ceremonial uncleanness and purification are explained to them, while the regulations governing sexual relations are also impressed upon them. On the whole, the instruction given must be considered decidedly salutary and wholesome, though it naturally varies, no doubt, with the personality of the instructor. The performance of the actual ceremony will be found fully described and illustrated in my articles on this subject in *Man* of September 1913 and May 1915. After the performance of the operation a month or more elapses for the healing of the patients, after which there is a period of considerable sexual licence. Subsequently the initiate settles down as a normal adult member of the tribe and is in a position to marry.

After the wound is healed, and the patient has been shaved, another ceremony takes place. A goat is killed by an elder, and sticks of the Migumu-tree are gathered and placed on the ground about two paces in front of the parents' hut; on these sticks the carcase of the goat is placed. The parents then sit outside the door and the child stands with its back to the goat. He (or she) then steps over it backwards, takes it up, puts it at the feet of the parents, and then goes into the hut, keeping silent throughout. The parents then follow, and all three eat the meat of the goat, while from the skin are cut three strips to form *Rukwara*, in the form of a finger-ring for the father, an anklet for the mother, and a strip, worn bandolier-fashion, for the child. These are worn for three days, and are then thrown under the wearer's bed—but this detail is uncertain.

There is a widespread tendency for the age of circumcision to be lowered; the fact that it adds somewhat to the dignity of the father perhaps encourages this, while, of course, the young people themselves are anxious to become officially " grown-up." Since there is no longer the necessity for the initiated boy to take his place at once as a warrior, that former objection has disappeared; consequently, one sometimes sees quite young boys who are considered ready for initiation, and there is a similar tendency among the girls. This is very much to be deplored, as such precocity must be most harmful; the object of the ancient custom is to provide a definite entrance to the duties and functions of adult life and sexual matters: the reduction in age, therefore, must be very demoralizing. The view that poll-tax becomes payable as soon as a boy is initiated, and that adult work may then be expected from him, may have some effect in stopping this unfortunate tendency, which is certainly deplored by the best element among the natives.

The ceremony has frequently been attacked by ignorant and prejudiced peisons as being a direct incentive to immorality. This, however, is a gross misrepresentation, for its whole tendency is to regulate and legalize sexual relations. The fact that considerable licence follows it, is merely the result of the general lax native standard of morality according to European ideas. It is a subject which is not easily investigated, though nothing but the fullest personal inquiry, not only into the ceremony itself, but also into the preliminaries, will justify the expression of an opinion. It is very certain that ignorant meddling with this well-established and highly important custom can only be attended with serious results.

Ear-piercing.—This is carried out after circumcision, for the boys, the lobe of the ear being pierced by a doctor with an awl a few days after the ceremony, for which attention the father pays a pot of beer. A thin stick is first inserted, and the aperture is gradually spread, by means of larger pieces of wood, until it is big enough to receive quite large wooden disks; or a fancy article, such as a meat-extract jar, may be worn. It seems likely that the extreme distension of the lobe is copied from the Masai: the more primitive people are content with much smaller lobes. The upper rim of the ear is also pierced in several places, and sticks, quills or beads are often worn there; this, however, is largely a matter of taste, and the holes can be bored at any time, by a friend. The girls' ears are similarly pierced after initiation, though a small iron ear-ring is usually all that is worn: the heavy brass ornament of the Masai woman is quite foreign to the Embu tribes.

CHAPTER VIII

Marriage

THE young man usually contemplates matrimony as soon as he is full grown, though the necessity for the dowry payment may delay matters; it is, however, quite exceptional to find a man still a bachelor when past early manhood. Marriages are, on the whole, usually from inclination: the general equality of status makes this much simpler, and only the discussion of the dowry payment affects the views of the lady's parents.

The exact course of the transaction varies somewhat in each section: the following account is more or less the method of the Ndia Kikuyu and the Embu.

Should a young man see a girl who takes his fancy, he invites a friend, who dresses himself out in all obtainable finery, as does the lover. In the evening they go to see the lady and the lover proposes, to be referred to the lady's father should she be favourable. The next day but one they go to the father, who has been warned of their coming. The lady has prepared porridge and snuff; this is consumed, and the lover returns home. He repeats the visit next day, with a considerable quantity of beer as a present. The following day the men of his village go with his father to call on the lady's father, and on the next day the lover again goes to call, and takes porridge with the lady. That night her mother lights a special fire on the hearth, slacking it to keep it alight all night. The next day the lover goes with the dowry payment in cattle and goats. A goat is killed and the lady and her parents eat the meat, except the right fore-leg, which is eaten by the lover and the best man. He returns home, and repeats the visit the next day, with some more beer, after which he returns home with his bride.

The payment mentioned above is not final, as there should be further payments on the birth of the first and subsequent children. If the woman proves to be unfertile no further payments are necessary. This fertility payment is complicated and elusive, and a great source of disputes and long-standing debts; in some cases the claim may be maintained by the father's family for ten or even twenty years.

The Chuka marriage formalities differ sufficiently from the above for it to be perhaps worth while to give the detail at length.

The question of the marriage settlement is the business of the respective fathers. The actual decision to get married rests with the young man and the girl.

The warrior having reached an age when he considers himself ripe for matrimony—probably twenty or so, though the age varies greatly—he looks round him for an attractive maiden. After a few interviews, casual or premeditated, in daily life or at dances and

other social functions, the couple make up their minds
that they are suited to each other. The girl has no
hesitation in repulsing the young man if she has already
lost her heart, or if she does not care for him, but in
most cases the lady seems to be easily satisfied, and
well enough pleased with the attentions of the young
man to be quite ready to accept his proposal.

The young man then goes to his father, who takes
the first formal step by sending a present of liquor
to the girl's father; subsequently the old men meet
and discuss the matter, settling a suitable amount to
be paid to the bride's father. This " dowry " is then
paid over.

As soon as this is done, the warrior in the evening
sends a boy and a girl to the girl; they sit down in the
village, the parents of the girl knowing the purpose
of the visit; she is fetched and her father gives her a
goat " to grease her skin and face, to make her attractive," and she is sent off with the two children, who
carry her mat, cooking-pots, household utensils, etc.
On arrival at the village of her relations-in-law, she
waits at the gate till the father-in-law has presented
her with another goat. She then comes in and goes to
the young man at once, and they take possession of
their hut, the transaction being complete.

This hut is a new one specially built after consulta-
tion with a *mganga* (doctor) who has indicated a
favourable place to build it; this refers to the locality
and time of building only; the details of the hut and
the position of the door do not matter. The same

Periods of Life

wise man has also previously provided charms to be worn by the bride and bridegroom, such as armlets, anklets, etc.

The above describes the correct and normal course of the negotiations; but very frequently there are various complications. Of these the commonest is the poverty of the would-be bridegroom, which necessitates a debt being contracted which may well go on for an almost indefinite period; in such a case the bridegroom, having got his wife and settled down in comfort, is naturally reluctant to part with the rest of the price; in addition, not only do the original cows and goats remain due, but any increase that may take place during the delay must be reckoned in the debt. Conditions are also added sometimes making the bargain depend on the sex of the next calf of some cow; or a long-standing debt due from some other party is sometimes handed on; all such complications are naturally sources of constant dispute and quarrelling, and it is scarcely to be wondered at that the native Elders' Council is perpetually engaged in hearing such matters.

Head-shaving.—As a couple get older, and their children grow up, they attain the position of elders. As soon as the eldest boy is circumcised, the parents shave their heads, and continue to do so until their death. In some cases this is not done very regularly, and occasionally one may meet with old men who have quite a crop of grey hair; but as a rule the old people have practically clean-shaven heads.

This practice is not, however, confined to the elders;

it forms part of many purification ceremonies, as well as treatment for disease, while young men also shave off their hair in patterns occasionally (this, however, seems to be quite an alien habit). The actual removal of the hair must be a most painful process, for it is done with an ordinary knife sharpened up for the purpose, while sometimes a piece of broken glass may be substituted. The hair is damped from time to time, but no other preparation is made, with the result that the scraping of the skin is quite apt to draw blood. The patient stands the operation very stoically; but the need for better implements is quite appreciated, as will be readily discovered by the offer of an old safety-razor blade.

The wearing of the hair in a greasy pigtail, Masai fashion, is quite popular with the young warriors; but this would seem to be an innovation from the Masai and the Meru.

Death

Curiously little importance is attached to death, or to the disposal of the corpse; in fact, it would seem to be the least regarded of all the incidents of life. The main feature is the uncleanness caused by the dead body, and the consequent complications.

Corpses are almost invariably disposed of by being deposited in the bush, where the hyenas and carrion-feeders generally dispose of the remains. This somewhat gruesome method is fairly reliable under all ordinary circumstances, since Nature's undertakers are numerous and active; occasionally, however, unusual mortality will overtax the resources of the local hyenas, and distressing results arise (I have a vivid recollection of finding a considerable portion of a dead woman just outside my house one morning). Very occasionally, old people are buried; but I never heard of this being done in the case of any elder whom I knew. Indeed, many natives will deny that it is ever done, and I am inclined to believe that burial is really alien to the Embu tribes, though it is occasionally practised by the neighbouring Kikuyu.

Since the dead body is unclean, its presence entails considerable complications; the hut in which the death takes place must be destroyed, and the person who drags out the body into the bush must go through purification. In consequence, there is a tendency to build a small temporary hut just outside the village for a patient whose life is despaired of: a proper supply of food and drink is provided, and the sufferer is not abandoned, but the arrangement is naturally a somewhat cold-blooded one to European ideas. On the whole, however, cases of neglect are rare, and I have often known of patients who recovered after they had been taken out of the village to die: a conclusive proof that they had not been simply abandoned. Indeed, it is quite possible to find an astonishing degree of toleration and humanity shown to some wretched creature who is helpless and repulsive from an advanced condition of leprosy or syphilis; it might, indeed, be better from the point of view of sanitation and hygiene if the natives were rather more particular about infection and disease.

When a death occurs, one relative must drag out the corpse to the bush: in the case of a child, it is done by the mother; an adult is disposed of by the available next-of-kin, usually the brother in the case of a man, or the son in the case of an elder, though a wife may perform the necessary act for her husband. A woman's body is usually disposed of by her husband or son; but there does not seem to be a very rigid rule in these cases.

The possessions of the deceased need not be destroyed, though this is sometimes done with certain weapons or implements. The hut in which death took place must be broken down, however, and left to decay. The village generally is not affected, nor does any sort of *tapu* seem to follow, such as avoidance of the name of the deceased, etc. I was able to observe the circumstances attending the deaths of several important and respected people, and in every case I was much astonished at the very slight amount of attention paid to the occurrence. Mourning is hardly observed, though head-shaving and face-painting may be practised, to a limited extent, in the deceased's household. There seems to be no idea of the return of the spirit for good or bad purposes, and, indeed, the whole theory of ghosts is quite alien in Embu. There is a general idea, however, that a wizard might make some evil use of a dead body, and any interference with one, or even with a skull, is therefore regarded with great suspicion.

Periods of Life

One may occasionally hear a reference to the " Spirits of the Elders " or to some theory that ancient forbears took some other form after death; but such theories are very vague and, for practical purposes, negligible. The whole circumstances of death serve to support the view that the Embu natives have very little idea of any future life; there is certainly no accepted theory of any activities beyond the grave, and any question on this point always produced a flat denial. Nevertheless, in conversation with intelligent and thoughtful people, I have known them admit that the complete cessation of all activity in the case of the death of an active man was curious, and even unlikely; I never, however, obtained any surmise as to what the deceased might be likely to do, in some new sphere.

This materialistic outlook is a great stumbling-block to missionaries of Christianity and Islam; the ordinary native is at first attracted and fascinated by the accounts of some future life, but the lack of obvious and verifiable communication between the living and dead soon makes him return to an attitude of scepticism towards the theory of human immortality. This frame of mind is of some considerable importance in the consideration of native psychology, and I believe it to be much more deeply rooted than is generally admitted; it probably goes far to explain the attitude of cynicism towards any religious system which is so characteristic of the more sophisticated native.

CHAPTER IX

Food & Drink

THE food of the minor tribes of Kenya is mainly vegetarian, like that of the Akikuyu; but they also eat wild animals to a considerable extent. The variety is much greater than appears at first, and on the whole the dietary may be said to be generous, except for certain conspicuous defects. Very little meat is eaten, owing to the general poverty in live stock, and salt is as a rule quite a luxury. No fruit except bananas is eaten in any quantity, though various wild fruits exist, and are utilized when met. Green food also is somewhat lacking, as it is restricted to certain crops when nearly ripe, nothing of the nature of cabbage or lettuce being used. Pumpkins are eaten by certain sections, while sugar-cane is eaten raw; but on the whole the diet of the people consists of dry maize, beans or millet, usually cooked by boiling.

This appears to be the cause of a great deal of the skin and blood troubles which are so very common; certainly as the use of salt grows more general, owing to the sale of it at the local shops, the percentage of people who are more or less crippled by sores seems to

Domestic

grow perceptibly less; while men who have for some reason been subjected to a regular diet which includes salt (prisoners, workmen, etc.) are usually distinctly above the average in health in such details. Unfortunately the natives are very conservative, and it is almost impossible to induce them to try such things as cabbage, though European potatoes are growing popular, owing mainly to their keeping qualities.

The proportions of the various foodstuffs vary considerably in the different sections, owing to the local possibilities in the way of crops. Chuka, which is a very poor maize country, produces a quantity of beans in great variety, and these are, therefore, eaten by the local population almost to the exclusion of anything else. In the lower country millet in its various forms does well, and thus enters largely into the menu; but those parts which produce maize seem to be utilized chiefly for that.

All sections eat maize, beans, sweet potatoes, yams, sugar - cane and bananas; while some add millet, pumpkins and various minor items, when they are obtainable. Every tribe eats game to some extent, though there is a tendency to regard this as somewhat discreditable among natives who have come much into contact with Akikuyu; and some draw the line at animals considered delicacies by others.

The most omnivorous of all are the Chuka; these, unless sophisticated by contact with their neighbours, will eat practically every kind of animal, not excluding

Domestic

hyena and monkey, though these are usually acceptable
only to the old men, who seem less fastidious than other
people. Snakes are not eaten, nor are birds, though
boys may eat the latter until the age of circumcision.
This prohibition includes chickens and eggs, and a
warrior would be greatly upset were he to find that
he had inadvertently eaten something containing eggs;
the result of such food is to turn the offender bald and
pink, "like a European," and it is carefully avoided.
Fish also is regarded as inedible, because "it is like a
snake." Locusts are a great delicacy, while the boys
are very fond of flying ants, which are eaten alive, in
handfuls.

The Mwimbe are not quite so catholic in their tastes,
but still far more so than the Akikuyu. They do not
eat hyena or monkey or crocodile, while the people
of Upper Mwimbe refuse to eat elephant, although
those in the lower country will do so. In other matters
they much resemble the Chuka.

The Embu observe the same restrictions as the
Mwimbe, but they will eat elephant; there is a
growing tendency, however, for the Embu to take
rather the Kikuyu view of all wild animals as food.
They all eat pumpkins, which are restricted in Mwimbe
to the women and the old men.

The Emberre are much like the Embu in their
food, but the perpetual possibility of famine probably makes them somewhat broad-minded as to
restrictions.

All sections refuse eggs and fish, and birds are boys'

Domestic

food, as are also ants in most cases. Blood is drawn from the living bull by means of a stopped arrow, and this is caught in a bowl and mixed with gruel or other food, or occasionally drunk warm; it is considered very strengthening for invalids, for which purpose it is also sometimes mixed with milk. There seems to be a prejudice against certain beans as food for the warriors, and this is especially noticeable in Mwimbe.

All sections refuse to drink milk at the same time that they are eating meat; if any meat has been eaten, the subsequent drinking of milk will produce spots on the cow and calf. Three months must elapse between meat and milk, but it is also possible to purify oneself by eating a small bitter berry named *ngeta*, which grows on a large tree.

The restrictions and prohibitions as to the various classes who may or may not eat together vary to some extent among the sections, but the general principles are the same throughout. The sexes cannot eat together. Old people usually eat by themselves, though old men may, on occasions, eat with warriors. Uncircumcized boys cannot eat with any other class, nor can young girls. It is usually the duty of the woman to prepare the food, though in the absence of a woman a man of the right class may prepare the food for his brethren. It would, however, be entirely incorrect for, say, a boy to prepare the food for a party of old men. These prejudices do not seem to have any particular explanation, and may be described rather as points of etiquette than as definite laws. Nevertheless, non-observance of them will make those concerned acutely uncomfortable.

When an animal is killed, certain portions are considered the property of certain classes. The old men are entitled to the head unless they waive their right; they also eat the liver and heart. The intestines are reserved for the women, as are the kidneys; scraps and bones go to the boys, though it is noticeable that they are usually pretty generous scraps. The marrow out of the larger bones is generally eaten by the old men. In the case of a bull being killed, the neck is the peculiar property of the warriors, while the chief expects a shoulder. It will be noticed that the owner does not have much voice in the disposal of his property, but he at any rate secures a good feed for himself and his friends.

The meat is cooked by roasting it on sticks over the fire; the skewers are long green sticks, which do not easily burn, and they are supported on forked sticks at either end, to make a sort of large gridiron; scraps are sometimes stuck on upright sticks in the ground in front of the fire. Meat is occasionally dried in the sun to preserve it, but this is not well done, and it does not last long: possibly this is a trick learnt from strangers.

Grain is generally eaten in the form of a pasty mass, which is obtained by boiling the whole maize or beans or millet until it grows soft; flour is frequently eaten in the same way, though it is not liked as a steady diet. It is made by a preliminary pounding in a wooden mortar, followed by a further grinding on a saddle quern; this produces rather a coarse flour, but it is naturally clean and pure. Into such a paste grains of maize are sometimes introduced to make a sort of pudding, which is very popular as a food for a journey, to be eaten cold before starting. On the road a yam root is the popular food, as it is so easily carried by a string.

Bananas are of several varieties, the commonest one being eaten roasted while green; another variety ripens on the tree, and is considered rather as a delicacy. Sweet potatoes are roasted or boiled, and are largely eaten. Sugar-cane is eaten by stripping the bark and chewing it, but the real use of the crop is for the manufacture of liquor.

Cooking usually takes place outside the hut; the utensils are few and simple, consisting mainly of a few earthen pots for boiling, with the stones necessary for keeping the vessels upright over the fire. A stick is used to stir the food, but no sort of spoon appears in culinary use, though the wizard prepares his medicine with a wooden spoon about six inches long. Leaves are used as plates when required, but as a rule each person eating simply takes a handful out of the pot. Meal-times are largely dependent on convenience, and so long as one good meal is secured during the day, other food seems to matter little. Something is usually eaten early in the morning, which takes the form of the leavings from the previous night; a meal is often taken in the middle of the day, but the chief meal is in

Domestic

the evening; this may be any time from sundown to nine or ten o'clock, since it very probably consists of beans, which take a lot of cooking, and are therefore not ready at nightfall unless put on the fire early in the afternoon.

Grain is stored in large wicker-work jars, which are made by the women; radiating withes are fastened together at a central point, and twisted ropes of fine grass are then wound in and out in a spiral; the jar when finished is ovoid, with a mouth about twelve inches across, the greatest diameter being some three feet, and the height about four feet; but the dimensions vary greatly. The jar thus finished is set up on a little platform of sticks, and plastered with mud and cow-dung; a lid is contrived, on the same lines as the body of the jar, and a little roof of grass shelters the whole from the weather. If the grain is not to be used for some while, the lid is cemented on with mud. This arrangement answers its purpose very well, holding a considerable quantity of grain, and keeping it fairly free from insects.

Cooking plays no part in magic or religious cere-monies, nor do there seem to be any traditions connected with it. No remains of middens are to be found, the nearest approach to such a thing being the heaps of ashes to be found near most villages; these seem to contain nothing of interest whatever.

Very little in the way of " relishes " or condiments is used, salt being practically the only thing; this is now bought at some local shops, though it is still to a

Domestic

slight extent obtained by washing the saline earths which exist in some places. Nothing of the nature of yeast is used or known, nor are any drugs employed to mask hunger; sometimes the leaves of a tree with a slight astringent taste are chewed, but this seems to be chiefly done as an amusement by old men. The bark of the red " cedar " tree is chewed as a preventive of fever, occasionally, though it seems to have no properties to warrant this use.

Instances occur from time to time of earth-eating, but they are always associated with an outbreak of ankylostomiasis, of which, of course, it is a well-known symptom.

Cannibalism is unknown and is regarded with the greatest horror; their neighbours sometimes accuse the Chuka of having practised it in the past, but even if true, this was probably only under stress of extreme famine.

The liquors employed are four: a watery gruel made by stirring up flour and water, and three intoxicating beverages. The last are drunk only on special occasions; the gruel is freely used as a food which is quickly taken; but nothing is drunk with meals. When a man is thirsty he drinks water, usually from the nearest stream.

The chief intoxicant is sugar-cane wine; this is widely popular, indeed too widely so; although in theory restricted to elders and ceremonial occasions, it is becoming undesirably common among other sections of the population.

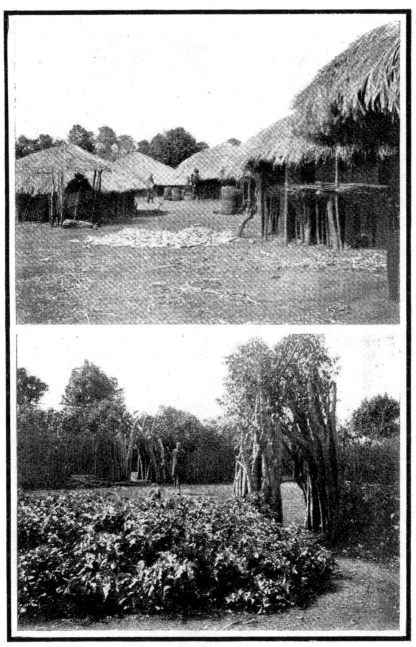

INTERIOR OF A VILLAGE.

In the foreground is a heap of mealie cobs waiting for the grains to be stripped off and stored.

ENTRANCE TO A VILLAGE.

Note the outer ring of thorn bush and the inner stockade ; the gates are closed by thrusting poles between the uprights.

Domestic

It is made by the women and the men working together. A quantity of cane is cut, barked with knives, and pounded in trough-shaped mortars made out of a solid tree, heavy pestles some five feet long being used by the women. When in a fibrous condition it is carried away on wicker platters to the men, who wring the juice out of it by winding string round bundles of it, which are twisted in opposite directions round a central spindle of wood; these bundles are squeezed with the hand over a gourd. The juice is then carried away in narrow-necked gourds and stood for a night in a hut, the warmth assisting fermentation, which is commenced by putting in a few pods of the alofa-tree; the next morning the wine is ready for drinking. Large quantities are made on special occasions, and some people indulge very freely in it, drinking as much as a gallon; they then grow noisy and quarrelsome, and a fight often ensues; generally, however, other people interfere to suppress the trouble. Drunkenness is not regarded with any special disapproval, though it is considered decidedly wrong for a warrior to be intoxicated, and much more so for a woman; but, unfortunately, such cases do occur, and by no means infrequently, especially among the people of Lower Mwimbe.

A beer is made from millet by a somewhat elaborate process. The grain is wetted and put into a pot; there it is left for three days until it begins to swell. It is then taken out and spread out in the sun to dry, after which it is ground and stored in a gourd. A second lot is prepared, and the flour is made into a gruel with water; this is warmed, and when heated through the original flour is added; the whole is left for a night, when it is ready for drinking, the entire process taking some ten days. This is usually made fairly strong, so as to be more intoxicating than the sugar-cane wine, but the strength depends upon the amount of water added to it. No sort of seed or plant is added to promote fermentation.

The mead is made by mixing strained honey and water, usually in the proportion of two of water to one of honey; this is left for a night or more to ferment, warmth accelerating the process, after which it is ready for drinking.

The Kikuyu name of cane wine, *njohi*, becomes in Embu *njobi*, while the name of the fermenting tree-pod, which in Kikuyu is *murátina*, is in Embu, Chuka and Mwimbe *murigi*. Millet beer is *márua*.

Distillation is unknown, and no record seems to exist as to where the art of brewing was learned. No special ceremony is attached to the drinking of liquors, though they always figure in any function, apparently chiefly as a means of entertaining the guests. A pot of liquor often figures as the payment for certain services or dues, or as a compliment to an elder—a custom which shows not the slightest sign of dying out as long as the elders have any authority !

No hot drinks are used, and milk is only sparingly drunk, and then under the restrictions mentioned above.

Domestic

Bee-keeping.—The most expert of all the minor tribes of Kenya in the art of bee-keeping are the Emberre; it is, indeed, their main means of subsistence, the honey being a local article of trade, and the beeswax having a considerable value in a civilized market. The following details are given as representative of the customs not only in Emberre, but also in other parts where bee-keeping is followed.

A large section of tree-trunk (if possible with the centre beginning to rot), some three feet long by a foot in diameter, is chosen and smoothed down with the little native axe; it is then laboriously hollowed out with axe and long-handled chisel, leaving a wall of about an inch in thickness. Two end-pieces are then made to fit the ends loosely, being secured by wooden pegs, and the barrel is ready for use. It is now up-ended over a smoky little wood fire, with *makari* (beeswax) in the fire; the box is well smoked, and then hung up by a rope in a suitable tree, the rope being any convenient creeper or fibre, though *mukwa* should be used if possible. With the barrel is hung up a bunch of "medicine," consisting of grass; this is called *ngondu*, and is obtained from a *mundu mugo* (beneficent wizard): the object of this bunch of grass is to attract the bees.

The box having been hung up, the bees enter through the crevices round the lids, and build the comb inside. The owner takes the honey out about harvest-time, when it is most plentiful. The taking is effected by blowing smoke—not necessarily tobacco smoke—

Domestic

in through the crevices of the lid, this being done in the evening. The bees go away, or get stupefied, and the honey is then taken, being carried away in a wood and leather bucket (*kisembe*) brought for the purpose. This done, the box is closed up and left as before, no provision being made for the unfortunate bees which have lost their store.

The Emberre know of no " queen " as such, but they recognize a large insect which goes into a box and gives birth to bees. No special reverence or affection is shown to bees, nor are there any ideas that bees have special knowledge of any sort; nor is there any custom, such as the English habit, of putting the bees in mourning for a death. Should the owner die, the box and contents become the property of the next-of-kin, like any other form of property.

Bee-keeping has always been followed for the sake of the honey to make a drink, but the value of the beeswax is only a recent discovery; previously it was thrown away.

The Emberre claim that they, the Theraka and the Lower Chuka were the original bee-keepers, and that other people have only learned from them.

The theft of a bee-box was most serious, being punished by a fine of a bull or eleven goats; repeated offences might result in the offender being drowned.

Bee-keeping is practised by all sections, especially by those near the forest, who specialize almost as much as the Emberre. If trees are available the box

Domestic

is hung in the air, but if no trees exist it may be laid on a suitable rock or propped up on forked sticks.

The elaborate ornamentation found on Akamba bee-boxes does not exist in Embu, though a man may put a private mark on his box to identify it.

CHAPTER X

DOMESTIC (*continued*)

Huts

THE huts in South-East Kenya resemble those
of the Akikuyu on the whole, though certain
peculiarities exist; the main principle on which
they are built, however, and the methods employed,
are the same in both cases. The workmanship is usually
much inferior, and the size of the houses is decidedly
smaller, this being most noticeable in Chuka. There
is much more effort to conceal the houses in Chuka,
and they are often built near a thicket, or among bushes,
which serves to conceal the low, unobtrusive roof so
well that it is often possible almost to walk over a hut
before one sees it. The good-sized villages to be found
in the Kikuyu country are rare in Embu, and still more
so in Chuka; they are to be found, and there is a
tendency to adopt them more, but as a rule the huts
are in small groups containing four or five living-houses
only, and often less, while isolated houses are sometimes
met.

The framework of the hut consists of a circle of
poles sunk into the ground, leaving about three feet
above it; this carries a ring of pliable rods, on which
is reared the roof, which consists of a framework of

Domestic

poles joined together by a circle of woven creepers at the centre. If the hut is a big one, there may be one or more poles inside to support the roof. The size of the huts built varies so surprisingly that it is hardly possible to do more than generalize over such details. The roof is woven into a web with circles of withes, and the grass thatch is tied on in small bundles. In these details the construction is simply that of the Kikuyu hut, except that it is decidedly inferior in workmanship.

Certain peculiarities exist among the various sections: the Embu use a grass filling in between the uprights to help to hold the mud with which the walls are plastered; while the Chuka, and to a less extent the Mwimbe, use uprights which are much closer together, so as to form a continuous wall, by which means they eliminate the mud plastering altogether; but this naturally requires far more wood, which is frequently a difficulty. In the whole construction the only means of securing the various parts of the frame is by lashing them with twisted bark; there are no bolts, hinges or other fittings, nor do pegs or nails take any part in the framework. If the hut is at all large it is usually divided up by one or more partitions of plastered wicker-work; but as a rule the space inside is so very limited that it is quite impossible to subdivide it further. The Kikuyu " annexe " or outer partition for a house for the goats is not used; the animals have a hut of their own, or else sleep in the same place as their owner. No second storey exists, nor is there any sort of dug-out

III

Domestic

portion of the floor. A circle of stones serves to keep the fire in place, and to support the cooking-pot in wet weather; in dry weather the food is cooked outside.

Each person usually has a bed of a few sticks laid on the ground, with a skin or mat put over them; more luxurious people will have a small raised bedstead of sticks laid across bars supported on forked uprights. Children sleep at the foot of their mother's bed, other older ones being provided for elsewhere, either in separate huts or in the common hut of their age. Ventilation is not conspicuous, nor does the lack of it seem to inconvenience the inhabitants at all; smoke finds its way out, more or less, through the thatch, the door being very low, not more than thirty inches high or so, while windows are non-existent. The number of people who can live in one hut is surprising; it is not at all uncommon for a hut, some eight feet in diameter, and barely high enough to stand up in, to accommodate a couple of adults, two or three children, half-a-dozen goats and a few chickens; with a fire smouldering all night, the atmosphere in the morning is perfectly indescribable.

The door is a wicker-work frame, which is put across the opening and kept in place with cross-sticks inside. There are no interior fittings to mention, though a stool may be taken inside sometimes; a few convenient knots in the roof poles serve as pegs on which to hang small articles, and the various niches in the sides serve for the same purpose.

The building of a hut is not attended with any

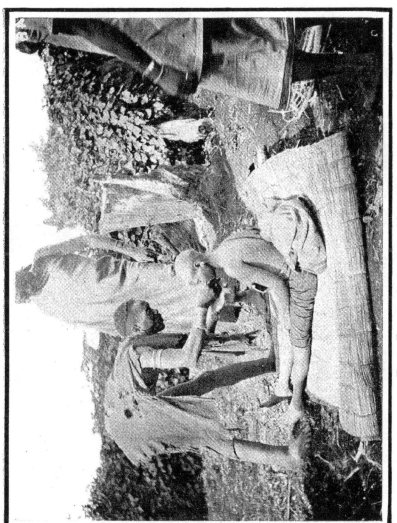

EMBU DOCTOR TREATING A SICK GIRL.

The goat's lungs are cut out, the Doctor inflates them and puffs them into the patient's face and afterwards into the dish of blood.

particular ceremony; if the architect has any reason to fear ill luck, he may ask a diviner to select a suitable day for the commencement of operations, and he may also ask him for his opinion on the site; but such measures do not seem to be essential. There is no restriction regulating the position of the door or other feature of the house, nor is there any special time reserved for building; no part of the hut is in any way sacred, nor is there any sort of spirit or ghost which inhabits the house.

The hut belongs to the builder, who is generally a married man; he has probably a hut for each wife, if there is more than one; the children sleep in their mother's hut, but unmarried girls in Mwimbe have usually a hut to themselves; old people have a small hut to themselves as a rule, while they occasionally go off and live by themselves in a little hut away in the bush—this because they wish to, and in no way because they are driven out.

The arrangements for the boys and young men vary considerably among the various sections. In Embu it is the practice for uncircumcized boys to continue to sleep in their mother's hut till they become warriors; after that they either sleep in huts of their own, or two or three will join in making a hut, which differs from the usual pattern in having a floor of crossed sticks raised off the ground, similar to that of a store hut; this is known as an *ikumbi*. They object to the idea of sleeping in a large general hut, owing to the danger of a night raid accounting for all of them in one swoop.

Domestic

In Chuka and Mwimbe, however, the *gharu* system exists : these huts are peculiar in construction, and play a large part in the life of the young men. A typical one may be described as follows :—The hut is built on the same principle as the ordinary one, but it is far larger, being some eighteen or twenty feet across, and ten to twelve feet in height in the centre, and four or five at the walls, the latter being of sticks placed close together and not plastered with mud. There is a stout centre pole, with usually six other poles arranged at the points of a hexagon round the centre, to help to support the roof; the general structure of the latter is the same as that of an ordinary hut, and the thatch is put on in the same way. About two-thirds of the circle are filled in with beaten soil to make a raised bed; this extends from the wall to the subsidiary centre poles, where the earth is supported by sticks laid against the uprights; the height of the bed from the ground is about two feet. At the head of the sleeper is kept his shield, which is placed against the wall; the spears are kept on the ledge over the door, formed by the roof poles extending over the uprights of the wall, which terminate in a woven band of withes. On the right of the door, going in, in the space left between the end of the bed and the door, are kept the horns or drums used for summoning the neighbourhood, and such bows and arrows as the occupants may have; there is also very often a board for the game of *uthi*. A few gourds and vessels are also kept there, and belts, swords and bags are hung from the wall. On the left side of the

Domestic

door is a circle of stones filling a gap in the wall, which serves for sanitary purposes; in former times the elders insisted on the young men keeping these stones moist by a method which necessitated the personal attendance of a warrior, a sort of rudimentary system of sentries being thus ensured. In the centre of the hut, between the main pole and the door, are a few stones to contain the fire. Such huts are generally very old, the timbers being black with age, and the heap of ashes outside being, in some cases, ten or twelve feet high. There is a stout hedge surrounding the hut, with a door contrived of growing trees interlaced; no other hut exists in the enclosure, which is generally close to a village. The details of these places vary surprisingly little, but as a rule the Mwimbe ones seem to be rather bigger than those of Chuka.

These huts served as a living and sleeping place for the warriors of the neighbourhood, and also formed a guard-house for protection against raids; but they were certainly also a trap in case of surprise: it is an easy matter to enter one at night when the thirty or forty inmates are sunk in the deep sleep of the African; the spears over the door can be secured and the sleepers are at the mercy of the invader.

A somewhat similar hut is occupied by the bigger boys in Chuka, but it lacks the military details of the warrior's *gharu*; some such arrangement is obviously necessary, owing to the later age for circumcision which obtains in Chuka.

The custom of building such places appears to come

from Meru, where it obtains on an even more elaborate scale, the name *gharu* being used there. The Akikuyu young men build special huts for themselves, but for a few only; like the Embu, these are floored with sticks, the name being *kithunu* or *singira*.

The average village in Embu is haphazard in arrangement, and there seems to be no rule at all for the position of the huts. There are usually from three to ten or more living-houses, with another two or three used for goats, and some four or five food-stores. These latter are merely ordinary huts with a raised floor of crossed sticks to keep the grain or other food from lying on the earth exposed to destruction by damp, insects or vermin. Round the whole group there is a hedge, not as a rule in very good condition, with one or two paths leading through gaps. No special provision is made for the protection of the water supply, which is merely the nearest stream; and sanitary arrangements are represented by the surrounding bush. No provision is made for markets, but there is sometimes a clear spot by the side of the road where people meet in a haphazard way to sell food. All the tribes of South-East Kenya are conspicuously lacking in such arrangements, and there is nothing like the large and well-attended markets at regular dates which exist all over the Kikuyu country.

Lake-dwellings are, naturally, non-existent, since lakes or rivers suitable to them are not to be found. No temporary structures which can be moved about are used, though chiefs take readily to the idea of a

Domestic

tent when they see one. Caves are practically non-existent in the locality, so there is no trace of cave-dwelling. Tree huts are occasionally made in which to spend the night in the fields guarding the crops or herds; they are mere platforms with a slight grass roof for a temporary shelter.

Cattle

The domestic animals kept by the minor tribes of Kenya consist of cattle, goats, sheep and chickens; the foxy, curly-tailed dog which is met with in such a large part of Africa is occasionally found in Kenya, but the keeping of dogs is not very general. Horses, mules and donkeys are foreign to the people, but they are appreciated by the chiefs and wealthier men, who buy them for riding purposes. Cats are liked, but are rarely met with, being quite foreign to the country. No birds other than chickens are tamed, though the natives would probably take to poultry-keeping with alacrity. There is no attempt to domesticate any of the wild animals of the country, nor are any pets kept.

The domestic animals seem to present very few peculiarities, and, except that they are rather inferior in quality, they are the same as those of all the sur-rounding tribes. There was, however, a breed of cattle, which has now died out, which possessed far larger horns than the existing breed, and are said to have been finer animals in every way. They are said to have been very numerous, and to have been killed off in the epidemic of rinderpest which occurred, apparently, about 1890;

Domestic

other accounts seem to throw some doubt on the date, and it appears more likely that the extinction of the breed took some little time. There are no traces of these animals now left except the horns, which are occasionally to be met with, made into drinking-vessels; these nearly always come from Emberre. These horns are short and thick, the total length having been originally some eighteen inches or so, in most cases, while the circumference at the base may be about the same, in a large specimen.

Cattle are used for milking and for slaughter; the blood is also drawn occasionally and used to mix with food, or drunk raw.[1] For this purpose a blocked arrow is used, being fired into the animal's shoulder; the method is very much that of the Masai, and there seems to be some reason for suspecting that the custom is really foreign in origin. Milk is used freely when available, but cattle are so few in proportion to the population that milk can hardly be considered a common article of food. The animal is milked into a calabash, and this is seldom very clean; it is usual to smoke the inside over a wood fire, and the rinsing of the vessel with cow's urine is considered a wise precaution against cattle disease; so, when purchasing milk from a native, it is usually as well to provide the receptacle and to see the milking done. Butter and cheese are not made, though the Meru in Northern Kenya make ghee or clarified butter.

The hair of cattle and sheep is merely thrown away; no sort of felt is made, and the hide is shaved clean

118

Domestic

when it is prepared. When used for shields, the ox-hide is left with the hair on, and the shield is completed before the skin is shaved, this being the last process previous to painting the design.

Goat's milk is not used, the animals being kept for slaughter only: this purpose is especially prominent, as they are required for all ceremonies, in addition to the food supply.

No use is made of any bull or goat except for the purposes mentioned above; no draught animal is used, and they do not appear in any way in connection with threshing or other agricultural work.

Cattle are usually branded, each owner putting on a personal mark; while the ears are frequently cut or slit in a particular manner to serve as a mark, this being the method of marking goats and sheep. The brand is generally crude, consisting of one or two straight or curved lines burnt on the animal's shoulder or hind-quarter.

NOTE

[1] " They can march for ten days together without dressing victuals, during which time they subsist upon the blood drawn from horses " (*Travels of Marco Polo*, " The Tartars").

CHAPTER XI

ALL the Embu tribes are clever at producing fire by friction, though the art is naturally rapidly disappearing with the introduction of matches. The principle utilized is the friction set up between a drill of soft fibrous wood working in a socket of hard dense wood. A stick some twelve or eighteen inches in length, and about the thickness of a pencil, is cut from some light fibrous wood and dried. Another piece of wood is cut, of some hard dense material, and shaped to about the size and thickness of the back of a small clothes-brush; the edges are rounded off and several " nicks " are cut in them. This piece of wood is held firmly on the ground under one toe, and the operator squats with the drill between his two hands, the point resting in one of the " nicks." It is rotated rapidly, the hands quickly rising to the top again as they reach the bottom of the stick. Friction soon rounds the " nick " until it becomes a small socket with a gap at one side from which the powder produced runs out in a little pile on the ground: continued friction increases the heat, until a glowing point is observed on the little pile of dust. This is half covered with a wisp of dry grass kept ready for the purpose,

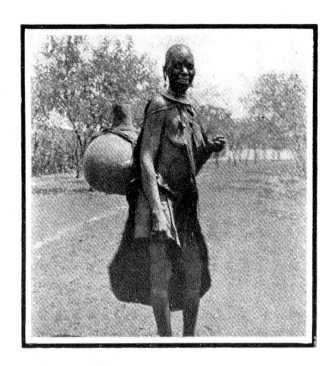

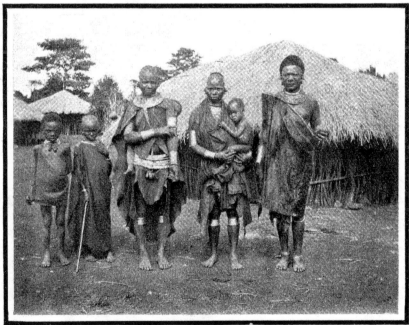

OLD EMBU WOMAN CARRYING WATER.

Note the shaven head showing her to be a *mutumia* (old woman).

CHIEF CHOMBA AND HIS FAMILY.

The Chief is wearing a cap of clipped feathers, and a well-greased goat-skin ; the ladies'
ornaments show Masai influence.

when a few puffs are enough to ignite the grass. The time taken is surprisingly short, when the two sticks are ready and thoroughly dry; after a little practice I was myself able to produce a light within a minute, under favourable conditions. The secret lies in putting a few grains of sand in the socket before starting, to increase friction; without this aid, blistered hands will probably be the only result. I have sometimes watched with amusement the efforts of Europeans to produce fire in this way, when they were ignorant of the detail of the sand.

The block and drill were usually carried with the arrow quiver, and the facility was very common.

I was never able to find that any superstition or reverence was attached to fire-making: it is not used ceremonially, nor does any sort of rite accompany the practice. It is usually practised by men, but I know of no prohibition on women using the fire-drill should necessity arise.

Traps.—The prevalence of wild animals makes trapping popular and necessary, both for the destruction of crop raiders, and for obtaining useful skins and meat. Naturally those sections nearest the forest are the most skilful and resourceful in this direction, since game is commoner in their area; but traps are readily made by all tribes.

Perhaps the commonest form is the game pit. This consists of a deep hole cut with perpendicular sides, some five or six feet long by two feet wide, and anything up to eight or ten feet in depth. This is dug in the probable path of the elephant, buffalo or other large animal which is expected to raid a plantation. The top is carefully covered over with sticks, leaves and grass, and the whole is dusted over to look exactly like the surrounding ground. The unwary animal which steps on it naturally has a heavy fall, and is probably unable to extricate the leg which is in the pit, thus remaining an easy prey to be dispatched at leisure. Smaller animals, such as pigs, may fall completely in, and be even more surely secured. To increase the efficacy of the trap, pointed stakes are sometimes fixed at the bottom, and I have occasionally seen these poisoned. Such a contrivance is so obviously dangerous that native law required each one to be guarded with light sticks set up near it, croquet-hoop fashion, to act as a warning to human beings, while too slight to deter an animal: the absence of these rendered the constructor liable for damages in case of an accident. Nevertheless, near the forest such pits are a real danger—I have a lively recollection of falling abruptly into one, though I was luckily able to save myself by throwing out my arms as I fell: my feelings, however, as I dangled over the sharp stakes at the bottom, until rescued by my spearmen, were far from pleasant.

Another form of trap occasionally to be seen in the forest consists of a heavily weighted spear which is hung in a tree over an elephant path: an ingenious arrangement of string ends in a line across the path, so that any animal breaking this receives the spear (which is frequently poisoned) in the back of the neck. This trap, however, is really characteristic of the Wanderobo, and cannot be regarded as native to Embu.

Bird traps are common, and often very ingenious : they work with a spring bow of tough wood, set off by a little twig disturbed by the bird when pecking the grain with which the trap is baited. A noose secures large birds, such as guinea-fowl, but a hoop of cane with a rough cord net over it is sometimes arranged to spring over and capture the prey in the case of small birds.

Rats and similar animals are caught by an arrangement of a noose attached to a spring bow, working in a suitable part of a little tunnel of sticks. The animal pursues the bait, which is scattered along the tunnel, till it gets its head into the noose, which is carefully hitched over points on the sticks so as to keep it open : as the points are all directed inwards, the least pressure on the string, inward, releases it, leaving the animal dangling by the neck. As fish are not caught, no traps are made for them, and the rivers are not the scenes of such activity as is the case in some other parts of Africa.

The practice of game "drives" is made use of occasionally, but I never saw any attempt to utilize long nets in conjunction with them, as is done farther south; in fact nets are curiously absent, for any purpose, which is the more surprising seeing how neatly string making and weaving are carried out. In this connection it may be remarked that there seems to be no trace of "cat's-cradle" or other form of string designing : the only form in which string is used for other than obvious purposes is the knotted lengths which are the usual method of reckoning a number of days : the headman of a gang will generally knot a string, or notch a stick, to count each day worked by his men. It was, however, an entire novelty when I introduced the tally-stick, and split it in two, so as to make a double record when the two halves were united for notching in the evening, a system which worked excellently.

Counting.—There is a curious system of indicating a number by means of the fingers, which is used to emphasize the spoken number : it is not done in the obvious way, by holding up two, three or more fingers, but is shown by placing the fingers in a certain way. The following are the details :—

ONE : The little finger of the left hand is pressed on to its palm with the right index finger.

TWO : Third and fourth fingers pressed by index finger.

THREE : Second, third and fourth fingers pressed by index finger.

FOUR : All four fingers pressed by index finger.

FIVE : The hand is closed.

SIX : The right little finger is grasped in the left hand.

SEVEN : The last two right fingers are grasped in the left hand.

EIGHT : The last three right fingers are grasped in the left hand.

NINE: All fingers of the right hand are grasped.

TEN: The closed hands are pressed together.

Above this, numbers are indicated by making " ten " first and following it by the smaller number; but the fingers are seldom used to indicate double figures.

The Embu tribes have a remarkable facility for mental arithmetic, and a man is sometimes found who can work sums in his head almost as quickly and accurately as a white man: this power seems to fail, however, when three figures are reached, and in that case elaborate calculations with bits of stick have to take place. There seems to be little comprehension of any number larger than one thousand; indeed anything over a hundred is rather bewildering to the less intelligent folk.

Measures consist of *kibi*, the hand (from finger-tip to wrist); *njara*, the fore-arm (from finger-tip to elbow), and *gwoko*, the arm (from finger-tip to shoulder). Greater lengths are measured by paces. Weights are unknown except for very rough estimates, such as "as much as a strong man could lift."

Games.—Hardly any games are played, even of the most rudimentary kind, and the children seem to content themselves with toys. There is no counterpart to the games of European childhood, anything of this sort becoming more of the nature of a dance. Little bows and arrows, toy spears and miniature bird traps seem to be the principal playthings. There is, however, one notable exception, in the shape of that widely popular African game which is played with counters in holes, and which may be described as a sort of graphic "Patience." It is known in Embu as *uthi*, and is a primitive form of the Swahili game *mbau* (board).

This is a most popular game with all sections of the Embu tribes; boards are to be found in almost any village and games are frequent. The game requires considerable skill and foresight, with a quick head for figures; it is surprising how well the most "uncivilized" natives will play the game; a good player will get quite a reputation as such.

The board consists of a slab of wood some three feet long, ten inches wide and three inches thick. In this are hollowed out two rows of square holes, rounded at the bottom like the cash receptacles in a till, to enable the pieces to be got out easily. At either end is a larger hollow, to be used for captured pieces. The game is for two players and the rules are as follows, roughly :—

Each hole in the two rows is filled with five round seeds about the size of a marble, known as *mbuthi*; should any seeds be missing, fewer seeds are put in the last hole, which may, if necessary, be left empty, and disregarded completely.

The players sit, one on each side, and each takes a row of holes and the right-hand big receptacle. The leader then takes up the five seeds in any hole and drops them into the next two holes, three into one, and two into the other; the second player does the same. The object of the game is to accumulate the greatest number of seeds. The first player now takes all the seeds in one hole and, working either to right or left, puts one into each hole, starting with the one next the starting-hole. He works to the end of the row, and then along his opponent's; when his handful of seeds is finished, he takes up those in the hole to which his last seed brought him, and with these he works back along the way he has come. This continues till the last seed in hand falls in an empty hole. He then takes up the seeds in the hole opposite it and puts them in his large receptacle; but he must " fall " or finish on his own side or he wins nothing. His opponent then tries to do the same. This continues till only a few seeds are left, when each player may be forced to waste several moves before he can score.

Should the seed " fall " in a hole which is the first of a series of empty ones, all the seeds in the holes opposite to the empty ones are captured. To score, it is necessary to invade the opponent's line and get back again, at least once. One " run " may last for several handfuls, and considerable foresight is required to see where the seed will " fall." The winner is the one who has accumulated most seeds.

A similar game is played by the Swahili, but with a board with four rows of holes instead of two, the game differing in detail from the Embu one.

The above are the rules which seem to be nearly those followed out by natives in play; there are, however, modifications and differences which are very hard for a stranger to follow; while the generally accepted legitimacy of cheating if your opponent does not catch you also adds to the difficulty of following exactly what is done.

It will be noted that the game requires a considerable amount of foresight and readiness in reckoning the exact result of any one move; one slip, and the move ends in disaster, just as much as a badly planned move at chess. A certain sort of special quickness seems to be developed in good players, who can see the best move almost at once, when the beginner is laboriously counting it up. The facility and certainty attained by even unintelligent natives is quite surprising.

Snuff-Boxes and Pipes.—Considerable ingenuity is shown in the manufacture of receptacles for snuff.

Like most Bantu tribes, the Embu are much addicted to the use of snuff, which is made by grinding up the dried tobacco leaves and adding thereto a trace of grease, the result being particularly potent. (Incidentally this preparation is very useful in guarding against attacks of biting red ants.)

This snuff is greatly used by the old men, though the warrior class are also addicted to it: a supply is usually carried in a small box slung from the neck by a light chain. The box is often made from a hippopotamus tusk hollowed out, or a suitable length of horn may be utilized; a piece of leather is sewn over the open end, and a plug, sometimes very neatly finished, closes the small aperture at the top, through which the snuff is poured out. A gourd is also frequently utilized, and, indeed, almost any suitable receptacle will be pressed into use at times ; one also occasionally sees a fancy article in the form of a wooden club, the head of which is hollowed out to hold snuff.

Much ingenuity and taste are displayed in the ornamentation of these snuff boxes and horns, and they are sometimes quite neat and artistic.

In Chuka, however, tobacco is smoked, the pipe being made of a suitable piece of hollow wood some eight or ten inches long by an inch wide. Dried grass and rolled-up tobacco leaves are stuffed into one end, to which a glowing piece of charcoal is then held. The pipe is passed round the group, each participant inhaling two or three mouthfuls of thick pungent smoke, which leaves him coughing and tearful, but apparently highly pleased. Much more neatly made pipes are to be found in which the wood is bound with wire, and a kind of rough mouthpiece is contrived. No special importance seems to be attached to the use of tobacco and no ceremonies are connected with it. The practice of smoking and snuffing seems to have been known from antiquity.

Iron-working — Chuka.—The Chuka metal-workers are scarcely so skilful as those of the Kikuyu, nor have they the same assortment of tools. A typical smithy may be described as follows. The hearth is a conical depression in the ground, sheltered by a thatch roof, but no walls. A large stone acts as a back to the hearth, and two smaller ones keep in position the pottery nozzle of the bellows. This nozzle is lashed to the leather of the bellows, which consists of two triangular-shaped flat skin bags. The short side opposite the nozzle is left open, and two sticks are sewn along the edges, and these have loops to take the fingers. The bellows are worked alternately, one hand for each, the hands being raised and depressed in turn. The hand rising opens the bag by means of the finger and thumb, which fills the bag with air. The fingers then close and the bag is compressed by lowering the hand, when the air is driven through the nozzle. Each bag is opened and closed about twenty times to the minute —or rather quicker, when a special heat is required. The bellows are pegged down on either side of the centre roof pole. The smith sits near the hearth while his assistant works the bellows. The fire is a charcoal one occasionally sprinkled with water.

On the smith's left is a vessel of water in which he keeps his tools, which consist of pincers or tongs, large and small hammer, one or two awls; while a small stone anvil stands at hand; for sharpening new axe-blades, etc., there is a large whetstone. A wood socket is also used for holding lengthy pieces of iron, such as swords, when only one part is being worked.

The forge acts well and gives a great heat: welds can be carried out very neatly. The iron is brought to sparking-point, quickly placed on the anvil and a sharp tap effects the weld. If, however, the spectators are frightened by the sparks and run away, the weld is a failure. Such a smith will turn out all the native utensils and weapons, such as spears, swords, knives, axe-heads, digging trowels, neck-rings, ear-rings and rough chains. These men are usually enterprising and intelligent, and will undertake considerable jobs.

An old pottery nozzle is a potent charm, and it is sometimes stuck on a convenient tree or branch, smiths in general being specially gifted in magic. These nozzles fuse and wear out quickly; I have seen a heap outside a smithy which measured ten feet by three feet by eighteen inches high consisting entirely of old nozzles.

Industries.—While the Embu tribes are mainly agriculturists and pastoralists, they do practise certain industries and handicrafts, some of which exhibit quite a degree of skill. They understand the working of skins, from which nearly all their clothing was formerly made. The hide is pegged out and dried, the hair is shaved off, and the skin is rubbed down smoothly with a suitable stone, and it is then worked up with fat until it becomes extremely pliable. The greasy and evil-smelling result is repellent to a European, but it meets native requirements very well.

These skins are often augmented with bead and shell work carried out very neatly and tastefully, the work being done with fibre thread and an awl. Beads are also strung to make necklaces and bracelets, considerable ingenuity being often shown in adapting seeds, nuts and small pieces of wood to supplement the ordinary trade beads.

Some little skill is also shown in carving, bracelets being very neatly made from horn and ivory, which are worked with very primitive tools, the result depending chiefly upon extreme patience. Small wooden and bone snuff-boxes are common, and sometimes show quite a degree of artistic skill. The most ambitious form of carving, however, appears in the wooden stools which are widely used and frequently carried by the old men. These may be ten or fifteen inches in height and perhaps a dozen inches in width. They are usually circular and four-legged, being carved out of a solid block. The designs vary considerably and are usually enhanced with patterns and shading burned into the wood, the final result being sometimes quite artistic. Very great patience is necessary for the construction of one of these stools, but even more is required for the hollowing out of the wooden mortar used in grinding corn. In this case a solid section of tree-trunk, some three feet long, is laboriously hollowed out for two-thirds of its length by means of a long-handled chisel, the outside being subsequently given a waist and foot so as to leave it vase-shaped. The hollow bee-boxes suspended in the trees also show quite a degree of skill.

The women are clever at working up fibre string into various forms, particularly as bags. These are made on the same principle as a grass woven basket, and may be of almost any size from a purse to a sack. They are very strong and useful, and play an important part in the women's life. Some attempt at ornamentation is made, the fibre being stained with vegetable dyes so as to produce bands of colour.

Arts & Crafts

Another form of industry among the women is the manufacture of grass mats, which they plait neatly also, with alternating bands of colour. These are used for sleeping on, and are also rolled round the baggage for a journey as a kind of hold-all.

A primitive type of pottery vessel is also made, though this work is limited to some of the older women. No kind of wheel is used, and the vessels are built up in two pieces, being subsequently joined round the centre-line and afterwards smoothed off with wet fingers. The firing is crude and not very successful, no sort of glaze being attempted. The form is almost entirely restricted to gourd-shaped vessels of various sizes. These serve to hold water and occasionally food, and will stand a reasonable amount of hard wear. Very little attempt at ornamentation is made, though sometimes a criss-cross pattern runs in a line round the neck.

CHAPTER XII

Dress

THE dress of all sections is, generally speaking, very much that of the Kikuyu and the Meru, but considerable modifications do exist. Clothing, as a whole, is decidedly scanty, the men, in fact, being dressed in a way that hardly satisfies European standards of decency. The materials used for dress in pre-European days consisted mainly of skins of various animals, supplemented with string and beads. In the more primitive sections boys and old men wore merely a waist fringe, consisting of a string girdle from which hung a line of strings in front and behind as a slight concession to decency. In addition to this a large square of goatskin with the hair on might be added, being worn under one arm and tied across the opposite shoulder. Various ornaments were, of course, also added. The warriors had a great tendency to adopt the style of dress of the Masai warriors.

The women wear a close-fitting under-apron of thin skin, greased to render it very supple. Over this comes a very scanty petticoat, also of greased skin, worked with beads and cowrie shells. The women wear no

Dress, Tattooing & Teeth-Filing

clothing above the waist. This petticoat tends to be more and more scanty in the eastern sections, until, in Mwimbe, it is the merest wrap about the hips, while in that section the second under-apron is not worn at all, a fact which has considerable influence in the matter of sexual relations.

The above description applies to conditions as they were on the first arrival of Europeans. All sections show the greatest readiness to utilize European manufactures to replace the skins formerly used; in particular, unbleached calico will be cut to the same shape, well greased and rubbed with red clay, until it bears quite a resemblance to the original skin garment. The women, however, appear to be much more tenacious of the skin dress, though this is possibly owing to the fact that their lords and masters usually reserve the more expensive clothes for their own use. In addition to adapting European manufactures to the native styles, there is also a great and growing tendency to adopt the principal articles of dress of the white man *in toto*. This is much to be deplored, since it not only represents the breaking down and disappearance of the salutary old tribal traditions and observances (as well as from the point of view of the picturesque), but it has also an undeniably bad effect upon health. A native returning from work at the coast will come back wearing a cheap cotton shirt, with a coat and pair of trousers of inferior khaki drill. These he wears morning, noon and night, practically until they drop off, to the inevitable encouragement of vermin among a naturally

135

Dress, Tattooing & Teeth-Filing

cleanly people. In addition, when travelling he may meet wet weather, in which case, on arriving in camp in the evening with his cotton clothing wet through, he will very seldom take it off as would a European, but, instead, will sit down opposite a blazing fire and consume his evening meal. Subsequently he gets drowsy and goes to sleep. The fire dies down and the cold night temperature eventually wakes him up chilled to the bone. The dangerous effect of such a practice upon a people liable at all times to chest complaints is obvious. Unfortunately the sophisticated native in European clothing can never be induced to adopt alternative sets. Any garment of which he becomes possessed is put on and kept on, even though the accumulation may be positively burdensome.

It is also noteworthy that the adoption of more sophisticated ideas in the matter of clothing appears to go hand in hand with the breaking down of ideas of morality, and this is still more marked in the case of women. A native girl who has discarded her scanty skin garments and taken to the more modern dress of the coast Swahili woman is almost always devoid of all moral standards.

Blankets form a very general addition to the men's wear, and are open to no objection, since they play very much the part of European overcoats.

Head-dresses vary to an astonishing degree. Masai and Meru influence is obvious in the case of the warriors, but the Embu tribes generally show con-

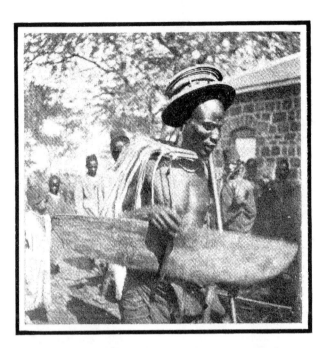

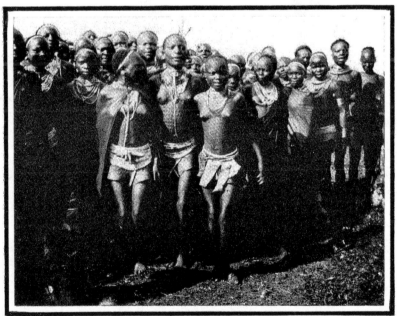

PITH HAT DANCE, EMBU.

The hat is made of strips of pith skewered together with thorns ; the tippet is of
fibre frayed out.

EMBU GIRLS' DANCE.

Note the pattern in cicatrisea lumps on the front of the body.

siderable ingenuity and originality in devising head-dresses for special occasions. These usually appear in the various dances, and they may be made of feathers, grass, various skins, or even worked pith. Further details will be found in the chapter on dances.

The shaving of the head is widely practised, and in some form or other takes the place of European hair-cutting. It is performed with an old knife whetted for the purpose, or, better still, a piece of broken bottle. The hair is damped with a little water and is then scraped vigorously off by a friend, on whose knees the head is rested, the patient appearing placid enough during what must be a most uncomfortable operation. This shaving of the head plays a considerable part in the various ceremonies, and is usually an essential of the ceremonial purification. On one occasion, in fact, I obtained important clues as to the identity of certain murderers from the fact that several warriors had recently had their heads shaved.

The hair on the rest of the body is also kept care-fully shaved, though old men keep down their beards in most cases by the pleasing process of tweaking out each hair separately with a small pair of tweezers carried for the purpose !

The shaving of the head is not as a rule practised by the warriors, who may adopt instead the partial shave of the Kikuyu or the matted pigtail of the Masai. The Chuka, however, are very much more inclined to let their hair grow into long ringlets, particularly in the case of big boys, who are given thereby a character-istically wild appearance. There is a tendency among the Embu for the warriors to copy the dancing costume of the Kikuyu, with the hair shaved right back from the forehead and twisted up, with cock's feathers pendent down the nape of the neck. This very unprepossessing mode gives them a lethargic, if not insolent, expression, very different from that which they have when wearing the Masai face fringe.

The use of grease as a body ointment seems to come from the Kikuyu and the Meru. The primitive Chuka do not grease their bodies at all (except for ceremonial purposes) and are, consequently, regarded by their neighbours as slovenly and rustic on the strength of this. The other tribes use oil and fat to some extent, particularly the warrior class, but the typical Kikuyu dandy, with his head dripping with oil and red clay, has no counterpart round Embu.

There is a characteristic style of dress worn by the boys when recovering from circumcision, and this varies among the sections, being either a cloth knotted tightly across the breast, under the arms and hanging straight to the knees, or else the same cloth, but with the ends brought under the arms and up across the opposite shoulder, to be knotted behind the neck.

The shape of the women's petticoat also varies to some extent, particularly in Mwimbe, where it is supplemented at the back with a triangular skin flap hanging down over the buttocks as low as the knees.

Dress, Tattooing & Teeth-Filing

Tattooing

Tattooing in the ordinary European sense is not practised, but cicatrizing, or the raising of scars in a pattern, is very common, particularly in Mwimbe. The skin is pierced and raised with a small awl and some kind of irritant is rubbed in which results in a pattern of raised scars. These are often carried out fairly elaborately on the women's necks, though no meaning seems to be attached to the form or pattern. This practice should not be confused with the marks left from the operations of a doctor who has made a series of small cuts or burns on the skin of his patient by way of a counter-irritant for headache or other ailment. This practice is very common and is widely believed in as a cure.

Another form of skin-marking consists in the application of corrosive juices of a plant. This is painted usually on to the cheeks in circles or stars. It blisters the skin and at first leaves bright pink lines. These, however, rapidly disappear, and in a month or two hardly any trace can be detected. No special significance seems to be attached to this practice.

Teeth-Filing

All sections of the Embu tribes are inclined to file their teeth. This is usually restricted to the two upper front teeth, but occasionally more will be operated on. The practice is by no means universal, nor do any rules seem to govern its application. A doctor, however, will sometimes recommend this being done in the case of a particular patient. There seems to be some ground for believing the practice to have come from the Akamba. It is carried out by means of a chipping with a small chisel, which is said to be very painful, as can well be imagined.

CHAPTER XIII

THE weapons employed by the Kenya tribes afford an interesting commentary on their martial history; in nearly every case they will be found to have copied to some extent the implements of their more powerful and successful neighbours. In consequence it is often difficult to decide what was the original form of the weapon under consideration, and how much it owes to quite recent imitation of Masai, Akamba, or other strangers.

The most obvious of these alien influences is that of the Masai, as might be expected; this, however, probably came through the Akikuyu, and not direct, since it is doubtful if the Masai ever came much into contact with the peoples of South-East Kenya. But they were so generally recognized as the most formidable fighting race in the country that their weapons and methods were copied slavishly by their weaker neighbours. The Kikuyu warrior imitated every detail of the Masai fighting equipment, even down to copying the designs painted on the shields, though these became meaningless when separated from their original owners. In time the same types grew popular and fashionable in Embu and Chuka, though they became

141

debased in the transition; the local imitations of the Masai spear were clumsy and ill-balanced when compared with the original.

It is possible, however, to distinguish to some extent between the older and the newer forms; alien influence is so recent that the changes are all quite novel, and a surprising variety of types is found in actual use.

In addition, careful observation will still detect the remains of older forms which survive in games and ceremonies, or in implements not intended for weapons.

A distinction may be made between the sections which seem to use the spear as their chief weapon and those who prefer the bow and arrow: this is probably to be explained by the influences to which each has been exposed. The spear is found as the usual arm carried all along the boundary of the Kenya forest; the use of the bow is understood to some extent, but it is not as a rule carried. In the lower country the bow is much more often seen, and it is not unusual to meet a man armed only with that weapon, though the spear is also popular. In such cases it is generally the small, light spear, and not the long, heavy Masai pattern. This is presumably owing to the Akamba—with whom the bow is popular—affecting the people on the Tana; while the Masai—who are responsible for the heavy spear—had more influence on the tribes near the mountain.

Throughout, the weapons of the Kenya tribes present surprising variations, and there are many points of considerable interest to be noted. Briefly, the present moment seems to be witnessing the final disappearance of various older types before a more efficient modern pattern of arm, though the two kinds are still to be met side by side.

Weapons of Offence.—Of these, the most conspicuous is undoubtedly the spear. This is the weapon which is generally carried by everyone who is travelling, or herding live stock, or otherwise engaged in some business which may necessitate self-defence. All men carry one, and the bigger boys who are employed to take care of the goats or cattle usually have some sort of spear as a defence against the numerous animals which might be attracted by the flocks. Women never carry them except ceremonially. The forms of blade differ greatly, and merge into each other in a way that produces an immense variety of types.

The form which seems to be the oldest is the little leaf-bladed one: in the most primitive forms this is about three or four inches long, by an inch and a half wide; it has a rudely formed socket, with a midrib running up towards the point; the workmanship is generally very rough, and the iron shows the marks of the hammer, while flaws and crevices in the metal are often present. This is fastened to a shaft about five or six feet long by means of the socket, which is quite short—not more than two or three inches—and close to the blade. The shaft is a plain straight stick of any tough wood, without ornamentation or any form of " grip." The butt is much the same as the blade, except that it is merely pointed, and has no edges.

Weapons & Warfare

At the opposite extreme to this pattern is the copy of the Masai spear. In this the blade may be three feet long by an inch and a half wide for most of its length, ending in a rounded point, while it swells out into two " ears " at the junction with the socket, this being about three inches long ; the width across the " ears " is usually not more than an inch more than that of the rest of the blade. There is a stout midrib running all the way down the blade, which is concave on each side of this rib, the final edge being given by sharpening the sides to a " stiff " edge. The shaft is of wood, very short, and only just sufficient to give a grip for the slim native hand ; there is very seldom any ornament on it, though there may rarely be seen a few threads of wire or a string of small beads tied round it. The butt is about equal in length to the blade ; it is rounded for most of its length, but in most patterns it is square for some two or three inches below the socket, and these square edges are usually indented with a row of " nicks " ; there may also be a rounded knob between the square and round portions of the butt. The whole spear may weigh as much as seven pounds ; it is a clumsy weapon, and in the imitation the good balance of the Masai original is generally lost, the spear being too heavy at the point. When well made, this is a formidable weapon, capable of being driven through quite a tough shield. I have seen a spear driven up to the shaft in the body of a man, and, again, in a leopard. It must be remembered, however, that the Masai, who mainly used it, rarely met a determined

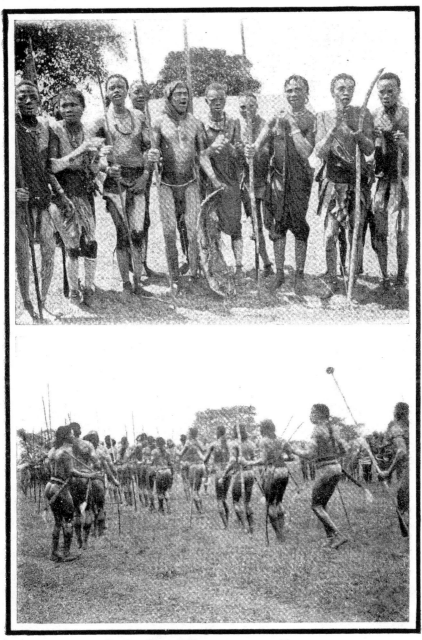

CHUKA BOYS' PRE-INITIATION DANCE.
The patterns on the legs are done with wet chalk.
MWIMBE WARRIORS' DANCE, A PREPARATION FOR WAR.
The performers wear no clothes, and carry spear stick and sword.

fighting man; they relied upon the first attack to defeat their enemy, and they would probably have found the long unwieldy spear and heavy shield a decided handicap if they had frequently had to meet such men as the Zulus, armed with a short stabbing assagai, designed for very rapid handling at close quarters, the length and weight of the spear bringing a great strain on the wrist if any real control of the point is to be achieved.

Between these two patterns an infinite variety exists; the little leaf blade grows larger and there seems some reason for saying that the old pattern reached its perfect form in a large leaf blade, some nine inches by five, of the same general form as the small one. This, however, changes gradually by the introduction of a shank between the blade and the socket; this varies greatly in length, and is often a foot or even more. When further developed, the blade begins to grow longer, while the shaft shrinks owing to the lengthening of the shank and the butt. This tendency continues till the spear is very near the Masai type, but differs from it in having much wider " ears," while the point is much sharper. The workmanship, too, is usually far cruder.

Curious oddities are sometimes to be met with: occasionally, in Chuka, a spear will be found having a blade at each end, instead of a blade and butt. There is also an occasional example of the Masai type of spear with the whole length of the weapon in iron, the shaft being indicated merely by two lines on the metal. This, however, seems to be simply a modern freak.

In all cases the blade and butt are attached to the wooden shaft by wedging the latter into the sockets; no sort of cement, binding or nail is used. The only approach to a sheath that is to be found is the small ball of feathers, fastened to a leather tip, which is slipped over the point in peace-time. This is a couple of inches long, and is often kept in place by a string running down the blade; it seems to be entirely a recent importation via the Akikuyu. Occasionally a strip of rag will be twisted round the blade, but this seems to be only a sort of copy of the feather ball. No instance is to be found of a spear with a tang in place of a socket; but it is interesting to note that the sword and the digging-knife both have tangs, and not sockets.

The spear, as has been said, is carried by most men; but a fully armed warrior carries also a sword, a club and a shield. He imitates as far as he is able the equipment of the Masai warrior, including the face fringe of feathers, the thigh-bells, and the general appearance and carriage, as he conceives it. But he is by no means a formidable character, and a very slight show of determination is quite sufficient to scare him away.

The sword is little carried and seldom used; it is usually worn by a man going on a journey, to supplement his spear, but it is of little real use, except for slashing creepers or bushes.

The types of sword differ slightly among the various

sections, the main variation being in the length. As a
rule the weapon is about two feet long; but this is
usually reduced to about eighteen inches in Mwimbe,
while the Embu specimen may be as much as three
feet. In shape there is little variation: the blade is
broadest about six inches from the tapering point;
there it is a little over an inch and a half; it then narrows
down towards the hilt, at which point it is not more
than half-an-inch wide; it is then finished off in a tang
which is fixed into a wooden grip—the metal is heated
and the wood is burnt away to receive it, no cement
or other means being used to secure it. There is no
guard or pommel, the sword being entirely meant for
cutting. Generally the sword follows the characteristics of the spear, with a midrib and double-edged
blade, hollowed on either side of the rib. The sheath
is made of two strips of wood scraped down thin, and
curved to form a hollow when placed together. Over
these is stretched a piece of raw hide stitched down
its length in the middle of one of the sides; a loop is
left on the other side, about three or four inches from
the top, which serves to take the belt. The mouth is
prolonged at each edge, to leave a crescent-shaped gap
into which the hilt of the sword fits. The bottom ends
of the wooden strips are rounded off, and the leather
cover is finished off by being brought through a chape
consisting of a metal ring. The name applied to this
chape varies surprisingly among the various sections.
The wooden grip is also covered with leather, which
may be sewn on, or may be a convenient piece from a

tail or leg which can be shrunk on " green " to avoid the seam.

The belt is of leather, about two inches broad, though sometimes considerably more. It has a series of parallel lines along it, made by a sharpened piece of wood while the hide is still soft; they run the whole length, and are about a quarter of an inch apart. The belt is fastened by a thong passed through a hole made in each end, to one of which it is tied; this thong covers the gap of some three inches between the ends of the belt, which is made too short for the wearer's waist. The sword is attached by the loop on the sheath; the belt passes through this, and the sheath is worn next the body, on the right side, with the belt outside it. When drawn, the sword is taken by the right hand, thumb down, and pulled out with a straight pull to the front, the point being swung upward; the motion is clumsy and inconvenient, the sword frequently sticking, and requiring the reversal of the hand before it will leave the sheath.

The belt, grip and sheath are stained a vivid red with a vegetable dye, but with grease and dirt this soon darkens to a dull reddish brown.

Knives can hardly be reckoned among weapons; they are usually carried in the leather bag which holds all the various items of the native equipment; they consist merely of a little leaf blade ending in a tang which is inserted in a wooden handle—in fact, a miniature sword. They are used for every kind of purpose, and, being of soft iron, they can be quickly sharpened when the job in hand requires a keen edge.

The axe, curiously enough, is a domestic implement and not a weapon; it would make a very formidable one, and would be handy to use, but cases in which it is employed as a weapon are quite rare.

Of all the arms carried, by far the most formidable is undoubtedly the club—that is to say, as far as results are concerned. It is probably no exaggeration to say that at least nine out of ten assault cases are carried out with a club; the weapon is always handy, it is very convenient to carry, and it can inflict a very serious blow.

As a rule it is cut out of one piece of wood, which may be any suitable tree; the piece is carefully selected with a view to a convenient knob of root or knot; it is then trimmed down with a knife, the final scraping being a tedious process, followed by a polishing with rough leaves which have the effect of sand-paper. The shape is a straight stick with a round head, which is usually elliptical, tapering up to a point; many varieties, however, are to be found, and the final shape depends chiefly on the patience of the maker. Various " fancy " forms exist, such as a hollow top with a plug, which is used for snuff; or a double head, with one knob above the other; while ornamentation may take the form of wire collars bound round the stick. The grip is not roughened in any way, nor is a pommel put on.

A curious form of club exists in Embu, which is composite in construction. A suitable stick is chosen, and on the end of this is fixed a round stone of about the size of a small orange. This is kept in place by strips of pliant wood which are bent over it and lashed to the end of the stick with thin string—three or four strips are usually employed; over this is stitched a piece of green hide, which is put on wet and pulled as tight as possible; it covers the stone head and the top two or three inches of the stick. The club is then put in the sun to dry, when the head is surprisingly firmly fixed in place. A small binding of string round the junction of the skin and the stick completes the club. It seems doubtful if this use of the stone is more than accidental—probably any equally handy weight would serve the purpose; no effort is made, as a rule, to trim the stone, nor is any particular kind selected.

This club is a most dangerous weapon, and quite a light blow is sufficient to kill a man; as they are made by all kinds of people, and not restricted to special artificers, they are very readily obtained. They may be fairly considered as far more dangerous than all the swords and spears in the country.

The club is sometimes thrown, but not, as a rule, with great accuracy; a small wounded buck or other animal will be occasionally knocked over with a club thrown at it, but this use of the weapon seems exceptional.

CHAPTER XIV

WEAPONS & WARFARE (*continued*)

THE only missile weapon employed is the arrow shot from a bow. This is far commoner in the lower country than near the mountain, presumably owing to Kamba influence.

The bow is a feeble one, made of a plain single staff, which tapers off into a point at each end. It is strung with twisted sinew, which is bound round each end, the bow being kept strung. The curve of the strung bow varies considerably, but is always more or less symmetrical—the stave is not pierced to receive the string, nor is any other device adopted to keep this in position.

The method of drawing and releasing is as follows. The arrow is put into position, with the nock on the string; the left hand then grasps the centre of the staff, the right hand holding the arrow on the string with the nock between the first and second fingers, and the thumb resting on the end of the nock; the bow is then drawn, held in an almost upright position, and to about two-thirds of the length of the arrow; the thumb is withdrawn from the end of the arrow, and the string is released with the two fingers. In Mwimbe

Weapons & Warfare

there is a tendency to straighten the first finger of the
left hand to assist in aligning the arrow, though this
is not always done. No sort of guard for fingers or
wrist is worn. The length of the bow is usually from
three to four feet; it is occasionally bound in places
with sinew, and strips of leather are sometimes sewn
on, but no attempt is made to form any sort of grip
on the staff. No case is used for carrying it when not
in use.

The distance covered by the arrow is about a
hundred and twenty yards, or occasionally more:
accuracy is very poor as a rule; the average marks-
man will miss a hat at thirty yards more often than
he will hit it.

The design of the arrows varies considerably; they
may be classed as wooden-pointed or iron-pointed.
Nearly all of the arrows made by the people of South-
East Kenya are poor imitations of the Kamba arrow,
and the latter is considered much superior, and commands quite a good price when sold. This arrow consists of a thin wooden shaft about twenty-four inches
in length and a little more than a quarter of an inch
in diameter; the point is V-shaped, and is made in
one piece, with a shank of iron some four inches long,
ending in a tang; this is inserted in a socket in the end
of the shaft, which is bound with gut or fibre to receive
it; in this it fits firmly, but not so fast that it will not
come out when the point is fixed in some object. The
other end of the shaft has a nock cut in it, with a sinew
or giraffe-tail binding to prevent splitting. Below this

is a feathering in three ribs, straight, and about two inches long at most; these are usually guinea-fowl feathers, though not always. They are kept in place by a fibre binding, while gum is smeared over the various bindings to keep them in position. A red vegetable dye is often used for ornament, in bands or dots, and the effect of a well-made arrow is very neat; it is difficult to believe that it is not the work of a skilled European.

This is the arrow which serves as a pattern for most of the tribes round Embu. Their copies are, however, mostly far inferior in workmanship, and the neat giraffe-tail binding, the thin, accurately made shaft and the finely cut point are all absent. The iron point is as a rule bought from a Mkamba; a rough shaft is fitted to it and a much cruder feathering is put on, the general design of the arrow being the same, however. But there is another type which comes chiefly from Theraka and Mumoni, in which the V-shaped point is replaced by a leaf blade, which is occasionally as much as two inches long; this is fitted by a tang into a wooden shank which again fits by a tang into the socket in the end of a reed shaft. This shaft is feathered in the same way, but on a larger scale, the whole arrow being bigger and heavier. This type is by no means so neat as the Kamba pattern, but it is a dangerous missile, with considerable penetrative power: I have seen several cases where these arrows were driven five or six inches into a man's body.

The other type of arrow is the wooden-pointed one.

153

This is considered inferior to the iron-pointed variety, and is used for hunting, amusement, or when the iron point is not available. The shaft and nock, with the feathering, remain much the same, but the shank and point are replaced by a wooden point from four to eight inches in length. This is sharpened at one end, and the other is pointed to go into the socket in the end of the reed shaft. This wooden point is generally cut into barbs like the hook of a crochet needle; these are made by cutting the wooden point triangular in cross-section and then notching the edges thus formed. But the point is often left plain, without barbs. There is an inferior form in which shaft, shank and point are all made in one piece, with a rough feathering and nock at the end.

The iron point is sometimes made with a small tang which serves to secure it to a wooden shank which replaces the iron shank of the one-piece point; this, however, is not strong, and is considered inferior to the other form.

A curious form of shaft exists, in which the socket to receive the shank is splayed out into points, which are kept open by interweaved binding of fibre, so that the shank itself fits into the centre of a circle of points, just like the handle of an umbrella among the ribs when closed.[1]

A stopped arrow, with a piece of wood secured to the shank to prevent extreme penetration, is occasionally used to bleed cattle; it is very similar to that used by the Masai.

Weapons & Warfare

Toy bows and arrows are often used by children, and the boys herding cattle generally carry them; these are merely small editions of the full-sized article. The little wooden arrows are used for shooting small birds, etc., but there seems to be no idea of training the young people in archery at all.

Very rarely a little bow a few inches long will be found in a wizard's equipment; it seems to be used for the dramatic indication of some person who has been selected by a lot-casting ceremony, for some reason. Little importance is attached to it, nor has it any peculiarities, being little more than a bent twig; any small stick seems to serve for arrow, being "filliped" at the person to be indicated. Slings exist, but they are never used for war. They are of netted string, and are used to hurl stones at birds molesting crops.

No boomerangs or throwing-sticks exist, the nearest approach to the latter being the club, which, as has been said, is sometimes thrown.

Self-acting weapons exist in the form of pitfalls, which are used chiefly for trapping animals, though they were, apparently, also used as a defence against raiding enemies in former times. These are narrow, deep pits, oblong in plan, some four feet long by two feet wide; the depth may be anything up to twelve feet or even more. They are covered over with twigs and leaves, and several sharp spikes are set up in the bottom; they are extremely dangerous, so much so that definite regulations exist as to the proper places to set them; anyone making one directly on a path or other place where a neighbour may be trapped is liable to pay compensation for any damage done.

Earthworks and forts do not exist, though all villages were surrounded with a dense hedge of intertwined trees, the only door being a sort of tunnel under the interlaced branches of growing trees; this tunnel was in some cases twenty or thirty feet long. The Chuka also constructed a somewhat similar sort of entanglement all along the border of the forest, by felling trees to interlace and form a dense thicket, which served to keep out raiding parties.

Huts are occasionally built in trees, but chiefly as a means of avoiding wild animals when sleeping in the fields, guarding crops.

Poison figures in the weapons of the Kenya tribes to some extent, though it is generally obtained from the Akamba; it is used to poison arrows, but it is never put on any other weapon. It is a thick black sticky paste when fresh and is prepared by boiling down the leaves and roots of a tree; it is the well-known poison of the Akamba, and acts through the depressant effect upon the heart. The efficacy of it has probably been considerably exaggerated, the natives stating that it will kill a large buck before he can travel a hundred paces. It is put on the arrows all down the shank and point, which is then wrapped in thin strips of skin to keep the poison fresh; when dry and hard it loses its efficacy considerably. Before shooting the arrow, the strip is torn off, leaving the poison fresh and sticky.

Quivers are carried to contain arrows, and are generally made of hide; they are about three feet long by three or four inches in diameter. The body is cylindrical, with a cap of leather fitting over the end, the whole being stitched at the seams. A strap passes upwards from the two sides of the quiver, on which the cap runs, and by which the quiver is carried slung over the shoulder. In it is often carried a fire-stick, with block and dry grass for making fire. It is often ornamented with beads, and little charms are sometimes hung on to it to secure the owner general good fortune in his travels; these seem to differ little from the similar things worn on the person. Another form of quiver exists in which the hide is replaced by bamboo, the two ends being made of hide, and the general design being the same.

Weapons of Defence.—The chief of these is the shield. This, like the spear, is simply a copy of the Masai shield: a wooden midrib runs down an oval frame of wood, on which is stitched a hide covering; the edges are bound with strips of hide, and the hair is shaved off after the shield is made. It is then painted in a pattern which is simply a copy of the Masai design; this is, of course, meaningless apart from the original owners, and no importance is attached to the particular one to be employed, which appears to be purely a matter of fancy. This shield-painting is still quite foreign to the tribes of South-East Kenya, and is chiefly adopted by those who have travelled about and have seen the Masai original.

There seems to have been an older pattern somewhat similar in design, but longer and narrower. In Chuka the shield is often very different in outline from the true Masai form, and old men speak of a still longer and narrower shield.

A curious makeshift is sometimes met with, in which the hide is replaced by tree bark; this is treated in the same way, and when covered with paint is difficult to detect; but it has, of course, little strength, and is used solely for show: the owner does not relish the detection of the imitation.

Numerous shields and boards of wood are used in the various dances and ceremonies, and their designs are varied and interesting; being in no way defensive they will be described with the ceremonies in which they figure.

There is one shield which appears only in a game—the *mkongoro*—which is an interesting example of a parrying-stick, of a fairly elaborate design.

No sort of body armour is worn, unless the heavy wire bracelet wound on to the left arm can be considered as a defensive measure; this is often worn on both arms, and it seems doubtful if its value as a guard is more than accidental.

Such other trappings as may be worn by a warrior are almost all merely bad copies of the Masai trappings, imitated by some man who has a not very clear recollection of the original; they are entirely alien

Weapons & Warfare

to the tribes round Embu, and are of very little interest.

Warfare.—The various tribes of Kenya cannot be described as naturally war-like in disposition ; there is no sort of feeling that war is honourable or desirable in itself, and when it occurred it was always for the purpose of obtaining some definite object, which was generally some sort of plunder. A successful leader was respected and admired, but more because he had secured some material benefits than because of his valour or prowess. If possible, the same results would always have been obtained by craft or fraud, for preference.

Such wars as took place, therefore, were raiding expeditions on the part of one side or the other. Whenever a real good opportunity seemed to offer itself, any section attacked their neighbours and carried off all the available property, which included women.

In such cases some acknowledged leader would get together a suitable force of young men, who would go to the local wizard for information as to a favourable time for the raid; this would be ascertained by casting lots. If the result was promising, the raid took place without delay. It lasted a very few days, and the party returned to their own country as soon as possible. No previous notice was given, since there was no question of any dispute to be settled; the attack was frankly intended for the enrichment of the raiders only, and surprise was therefore essential. Similarly, there was no question of a peace treaty or truce afterwards;

the injured parties contented themselves with await-
ing a favourable opportunity for a revenge in kind.
Occasionally there were attempts to redeem some
woman who had been carried off, by means of a payment of cattle, but such cases must have been rare,
for the visitor had no guarantee that faith would be
kept with him when he brought the stipulated amount.
Women captured in such affairs became members of
the tribe, and formed part of the household of the
capturer; stock was divided up by mutual agreement
—which was very apt to be disagreement.

Occasionally two neighbouring sections would make
a truce, by a general meeting of the elders of both
sides, who killed and ate one or more goats together;
such an arrangement was not very stable, and was
speedily upset, as a rule, by some act by an individual
of one of the two sides, which was regarded as an
act of aggression, to be followed by a raid whenever
opportunity offered.

There were very few rules of war to regulate the
behaviour of the combatants; everything seems to
have been fair, though there was apparently very little
purposeless barbarity; such men as resisted were
killed, and the rest — who were the majority — ran
away; all the women who had not made their escape
were captured, and all available stock was carried off;
but there was no torturing or maiming of prisoners
or corpses.

Women never took part in war, though there are
very rare cases where old women led the resistance of

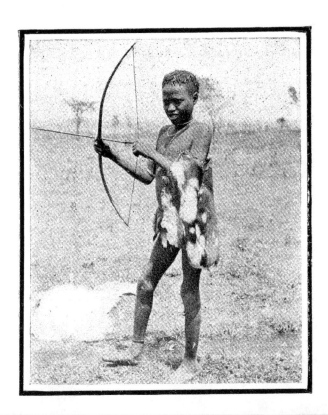

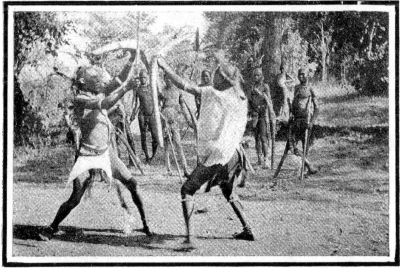

Mwimbe Goat Herd with Small Bow and Arrow.

The boy's bow is suitable only for shooting birds, but the picture shows the method of holding the bow and arrow.

The Chuka Shield Stick Dance.

Note the curious curved shield stick thickened at the centre to allow of cutting a grip for the fingers.

their people; as a rule fighting was regarded as quite outside woman's sphere.

Considerations of convenience in connection with crops and herds unconsciously tended to regulate the seasons for fighting, but there were no recognized times, nor were any particular areas selected or excluded.

Very little skill or organization was shown in preparing for war; an attacking party was merely an armed rabble, very slightly controlled by the leader, and defence was just the assembling of all available fighting men by means of horn-blowing and general alarm raised by anyone who happened to be in a position to do so.

The *Renda* dance, under various forms or names, seems to have been the prelude to a raid: the young men were apparently expected to do something in the way of cattle-lifting for the benefit of the community. But there seems to have been no attempt to lay down definite rules as to who was to take part in a fight; presumably the hope of loot was sufficient to induce anyone able-bodied to take his share of the work, while fear of losing property served to secure defenders for a village.

No sort of signalling was used, nor were there any words of command or drill formations.

War as such was undoubtedly detested by most sections of the community, though the more enterprising young men probably enjoyed the excitement; but all classes regarded it as a most promising way of obtaining riches, and it therefore remained popular with the more powerful sections, while weaker neighbours were forced by necessity for defence to keep themselves in readiness for hostilities at a moment's notice.

NOTE

[1] I was surprised at meeting a very similar arrow among the Makua of Southern Tanganyika.

CHAPTER XV

Art

IT may almost be said that Art in the proper meaning of the term is non-existent in Kenya; not only are there no elaborate examples of artistic effort, but utilitarianism is the ruling consideration in almost every form of industry, and in consequence even such things as pots and household utensils are practically devoid of any attempt at decoration.

There are, however, some details of native industry which may fairly claim consideration as a primitive sort of art, though in dealing with them it is most necessary to distinguish between local talent and that learnt from neighbouring tribes, notably the Akamba.

Personal adornment is the chief field for the exhibition of most taste, the bead and wire ornaments worn by both sexes showing considerable ingenuity and having sometimes quite neat and pleasing effects to European eyes.

Bead-work can hardly be considered as a purely local expression of art, since the beads are all imported, except for such seeds and pieces of wood as may occasionally appear in necklaces, etc. The method of using the smaller beads, however, shows considerable skill and taste. They are usually strung on a string,

163

which is then wound round the arm or leg as a bracelet or anklet, or the string of beads is sewn on to something as a base, usually a piece of leather. Beads are also used to work patterns on sword sheaths and belts, in which case they also serve as a means of identification for the article.

To a modified extent beads appear on the women's small skirts and aprons, though usually there is only an ornamentation of cowrie shells; these are sewn on in rows, alternating with the old-fashioned blue bead; or the design may be mainly blue and white beads with a shell edging. In any case the work is carried out neatly and the result is pretty enough when fresh and well executed.

Wire-work is also frequently used to ornament sticks, little collars of twisted wire being bound round the neck of a club or stick, very much in the way that many South African tribes do. This work is generally done by Akamba, however, and it may probably be considered as an introduction from them. In the same category must be placed the very neat and artistic wire-work on the stools which are often to be seen, carried by old men. These are, in all the best examples, the work of Akamba, though poor imitations are attempted by the tribes near Kenya.

Another instance of copying is the painting on the shields. This is carried out in striking and original patterns, painted on the bare hide with ash, chalk and clay. These patterns may, however, safely be said to have originated with the Masai, among whom they represent a species of heraldry. The reputation of the Masai as a warrior led to the copying of his shield, and the painting with it, though the meaning was thereby stultified.

The varieties of dancing-shields, however, are also decorated, and in these cases the design may fairly be considered as of local origin. Usually they take the form of a light ground on which are painted wavy lines in some dark colour; in the case of the long narrow shield the pattern is a sort of dog's-tooth one on either side of a central line. This is cut in the wood, and afterwards picked out in black and white. In Theraka a pattern of wavy lines is occasionally to be seen which is slightly suggestive of a similar sort of pattern found in the Bushman paintings of South Africa; but it is more than likely that this resemblance is merely accidental. The walls of houses may sometimes be given a coat of white chalk, on which are drawn circles or curly lines in dark clay, but this is rare, and seems to be merely a freak of fancy; no pattern or object seems to be held in view.

To the women belongs the credit of the work which is perhaps the neatest and best of any native product—the string bags. These usually have various colours worked into them by means of occasional strands of string which has been dyed in a decoction of bark; as the bag is made by working round and round a centre, a coloured strand introduced produces a corresponding band in the finished bag. These patterns are neat enough in a simple way, but they seem to be dictated only by fancy, or the string which happens to be available.

Some attention has been attracted by the so-called " picture gourds " to be found among all the tribes of Kenya. These are probably also Kamba in origin to some extent, though commonly made around Kenya now. In these cases, a gourd of which the skin is still not too hard to be scratched is marked with a thorn or awl with a series of lines, dots, circles and other markings, which are supposed to represent some story. The completed gourd is then carried by the owner, usually a boy, who rattles the seeds inside it, in time to a sort of chant. In this he relates his adventures, and the gourd is supposed to be the record of them; he will trace out a series of symbols explaining what they mean as he does so. There is no ground for regarding this as any sort of pictorial writing, however, since the symbols admit of no arbitrary equivalents; two different boys, or the same boy on different occasions, will give quite dissimilar accounts of the meanings. Possibly, in some cases, the symbols may come to have a fairly definite meaning to the owner, but as a rule it seems to be correct to say that they have much the same functions as the knot in the handkerchief of a forgetful European : they serve to recall to the owner's memory some detail which he might otherwise omit.

A little rough wood-carving is done, chiefly in the form of stools and sticks; but the patterns are very primitive, and the neatness of the result depends chiefly on the care and patience with which the work is finished off.

Art & Music

Music

The music of the Kenya tribes is primitive in the extreme, and their means of production are very limited. Practically, singing is the chief means of musical expression, and such other forms as exist might be called noisy rather than harmonious. The question of music is largely connected with dancing, from which it is almost inseparable in performance. The main characteristic of both is the keen sense of rhythm and time which is so striking in all native entertainments. The melodies themselves are simple and monotonous, but the time is by no means easy to follow, especially to one unused to the peculiarities of such music.

In nearly all the various songs there is a leader and a chorus; usually a recitative is maintained by some acknowledged performer, with a chorus of one or two lines which comes in at frequent, though not necessarily regular, intervals. This song may either be a well-known and popular one, or it may be a popular base upon which the singer embroiders an extempore running comment on any details that strike his fancy. A group of natives doing any combined labour usually select a leader who sings a suitable song, with a chorus in which all join, much as is done in a marching song, or in a sailor's "chantey" of sailing-ship days. The leader sings with considerable emphasis, and frequently rises into a most unpleasing falsetto shriek, from which he travels down the scale to the first note of the chorus, in which all join. Singing has a most stimulating effect upon all classes, and it is surprising how porters on the march will brighten up and quicken their pace if a good song is started. Equally, in telling a tale, certain speeches and dialogues should be spoken or sung in a definite rhythm; a good story-teller— usually an old woman—will sing each recurrent speech of certain characters in a suitable voice, in much the same way as an English nurse, with a proper sense of the dramatic, will give a suitable accentuation to the " Fe, fi, fo, fum!" which appears in her story.

The melodies are very varied and are in many cases quite attractive and " catchy "; well sung by a large crowd, with a suitable accompaniment of stamping and beating, they become quite infectious. The air is always on the black notes of the pianoforte, with one doubtful exception in Chuka, in which a suggestion of part-singing appears. Songs are altered in words and music fairly frequently, and the tune which is popular at one season gives place to another next year. It is usually impossible to find out when or by whom new melodies are started, and one generally finds them in full swing on visiting a village after a short absence. Certain tunes, however, seem to be regarded as so very satisfactory that they continue to be popular for years together, and even spread over large parts of neighbouring districts.

The voices of the natives are, as a whole, quite melodious, without the harsh nasal effect which is so trying in Indian singing; the songs are, however, so

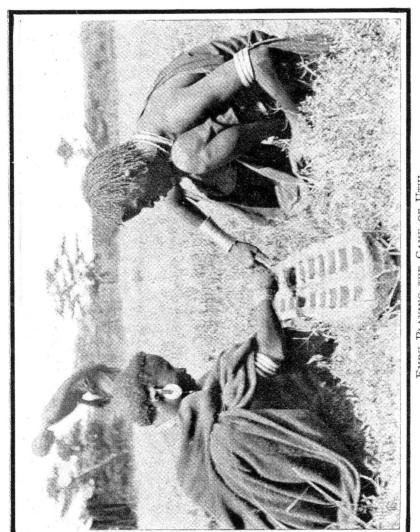

Embu Playing the Game of Uthi.

Note the long hair of the player on the right; this is characteristic of Embu and Chuka.

often struck up at such inconvenient times and with such maddening monotony that the European listener is usually unable to appreciate the performance. Certain ceremonies and functions have their appropriate song, which seems in most cases to be more permanent than the popular dance and working songs. Most noticeable among these is the song of the elders, who strike it up on arriving at a camp or village which they are visiting as a body. These songs are as a rule more monotonous and simple in character than those which are not definitely attached to any special function; indeed, many of them are little more than rhythmic chants.

The instruments on which the singing is accompanied are few and simple; they consist of trumpets and drums. In considering these, it must not be forgotten that the occasions when singing is going on are usually those when some assembly is taking place, and the easiest way to summon all concerned is by blowing trumpets and beating drums; so it is quite possible that the presence of these instruments at most dances is really only in a sense accidental. There is certainly no attempt at blowing a horn at suitable periods of the song, and if the performer keeps time more or less to the step of the dance he is quite satisfied. The drum is played rather more carefully in time to the step, but still without much knowledge of its powers.

The forms of trumpets are very varied. The commonest is one made from a horn, usually Greater

Kudu or Bongo. It is an interesting point as to how such numbers of these two rare animals were killed in former days, seeing that the first is absolutely unknown, and the second very rare, on the slopes of Kenya at the present day; the horns must either have been brought from considerable distances, or else the game has altered to a surprising extent in its distribution. These horns are merely pierced at the top of the hollow, so as to form a mouthpiece. Usually they are blown so as to give one monotonous and far-reaching note; but sometimes an ambitious performer will extract a series of notes from his instrument, though never in any definite sequence or tune.

Other forms of trumpets are made out of hollow branches, which are cut down and shaped till they are of very much the same form as the horns which they presumably imitate. Sometimes they are quite small, and can be carried slung by a string, much like a bugle. Some examples of wooden horns are obviously of considerable age; they frequently have pieces of hide shrunk on, the remnants of various magic ceremonies in which they have been used. Considerable importance is attached to such specimens, and they are kept in the top of the warriors' huts ready to be blown when occasion requires, as an alarm.

Drums are simple in form, and fulfil much the same purpose as the trumpets. They are usually made of hollow wood, with a skin cover, and they are played with the hand, by rubbing and slapping, or else with a small piece of stick. They are as a rule about two feet in height by some twelve inches across, one end only being covered. Sometimes a skin band round the middle is arranged so as to form a handle by which the performer holds the drum; very often, however, it is merely stood up at an angle and held with one hand. These drums are, like the trumpets, often regarded with considerable veneration, though for no very definite reason, apparently. They seem to play no part in any magic ceremony, except as a means for summoning participants, like the horns. To some extent they were used to give warning in case of attack, and they also appear at dances. But they are primitive in the extreme, and their use is very restricted; failing a drum, a shield or a piece of board will serve equally well; or in civilized parts a sheet of corrugated iron, or, best of all, a good-sized tank.

Beyond these simple appliances, no musical instruments are native to South-East Kenya. No stringed instrument exists in any form, and it never appears to occur to the owner of a bow to twang the string for the sake of the sound. Equally, no sort of metal tongue meant for twanging is made, although one might have thought that the many native smiths working in iron would have hit upon something of the sort. No metal plates or wooden bars for playing harmonicon-fashion exist, nor do the natives seem to find any satisfaction in striking a ringing piece of metal when they meet it.

As far as a taste for European instruments has hitherto appeared, "the mouth-organ" seems to be the popular favourite; concertinas are somewhat too complicated; penny whistles seem never to have been tried. But probably the real success in native eyes would be the "jews' harp."

Purely European and civilized music appeals to them more than would be expected; besides the enthralling fascination of the mechanism, a piano quite appeals to the native mind, in its musical capacity. Oddly enough, anything with a fairly definite melody appeals to them, even when there is little or no marked rhythm or recurrence of a theme; they speedily pick up a bar or two of the most unlikely music. Will it be considered a satire to say that certain pieces of Debussy are far more successful than any other music which has the same claim to be termed "classical"?

CHAPTER XVI

DANCES

THE dances are numerous and peculiar, and vary greatly with each section. Those for warriors have been largely affected by Masai influence in the West, and Meru influence in the North-East, the Embu warriors having a dance which is simply copied from the Masai. It consists of a march round in lines followed by the formation of a circle, when a leader sings a recitative with chorus by his comrades, accompanied by stamping. Usually a good deal of pantomime goes on, such as drawing of swords, lifting of spears, etc. The subjects of the song vary and are not necessarily about war. One popular dance has a recitative about the killing, cutting up and eating of meat, something in the style of the English children's song, *Nuts in May*, which runs: " This is the way we kill our game ; this is the way we cut our meat," etc. In this the sword is drawn at the correct point, the dancers sink on one knee, the spear is waved and so on, all at definite points of the song. When danced by good performers who know the song well, the effect is most attractive, especially if danced at night by firelight. Another curious dance is in celebration of the defeat of the Embu by the Europeans,

173

the song being an account of this with a refrain of
"*Mzungu kula ngombe*," or "The white man eats the
cattle." These warrior dances are far commoner in
Ndia and in Embu than in the other sections, but are
becoming rarer since raids and warrior dress for war
are disappearing.

Throughout all sections there are numerous dances
for young people. One popular dance, which appears
in various forms, consists of a line of girls faced by a
line of young men. The girls' hands rest on the men's
shoulders, and the men's hands hold the girls beneath
the arms. A monotonous song is sung, with interruptions of grunting in time to the tune. The girls half
spring, and are half thrown up by the young men, who
jump them in this way three times, when the song
goes on again.

There are also special dances for boys prior to
circumcision for all sections. The use of charcoal and
chalk is elaborate and characteristic.

The Pith-Hat Dance or Kiboicho of Embu.—This was
a curious dance for men of mature age, found only in
a small section of East Embu. The dancers wore hats
made of sticks of pith coiled round and secured with
long thorns, and little cloaks made of fibre dried and
combed out. A spear or stick was carried in the
left hand, and a crescent-shaped dancing-shield was
carried in the right. A stick some ten inches in
length was worked with the fingers upon this as a
clapper to keep time. A leader headed the two ranks,
led the song and gave the time for the stamping

Dances

and gradual sinking on one knee, which was all of which the dance consisted. This peculiar dance, with its characteristic hat and cloak, seems now to have disappeared.

The Mgiru Dance—Embu and Chuka.—This dance is for uncircumcised children of both sexes, and consists of the formation of the usual double lines, boys and girls facing each other, the dance consisting of a monotonous chant and stamping. One very interesting feature, however, is the use by the boys of the *mkongoro* shield-stick. This is a stout, curved piece of wood some three to four feet long, and about five inches wide at the centre, hollowed in the middle to form a handle with a guard. In Chuka this is used not only for a dance, but also for a kind of quarter-staff sham fight, in which the user parries with it the blows of his opponent's stick. Its use is restricted to boys, and it does not appear in war.

The Chuka Dances.—There are several dances characteristic of Chuka only, the commonest being the *Mboiboi*, which is for uncircumcised boys and girls. A circle is formed, in the centre of which a boy and a girl sidle rapidly round to the tune of a rather monotonous song and the tapping of sticks. The postures are obviously sexual in origin, though the dance does not seem to have any exciting effect or immoral influence.

A characteristic dance for old women in Chuka is the *Njeyi*. This consists of a circle of old women who move with a slow sidling step, one foot leading. The

Dances

arms are held up and bent at the elbows, and the body is swung from side to side.

A somewhat similar dance is the *Mbeni*, which includes a curious scratching movement of the feet. Both these dances are suggestive in the movement of the body, and are danced only by the old women of Chuka, other sections considering it improper for old women to indulge in such an exhibition.

The Renda Dance—Mwimbe.—This dance was performed by warriors and was an elaborate preparation for a raid. A small hut is constructed in the bush under the supervision of a doctor, who erects in the middle of it a bundle of various branches tied up with charms. The hut is a temporary structure, and only serves as a sort of central shrine. In the bush round this the warriors, sometimes as many as a hundred, go and camp for perhaps a month. There they live quite separate from the rest of the population. They strip off all clothes, but wear their ornaments and use a waist-band of wild sodom apples. Each day for some hours they perform a very monotonous dance in two lines on a sort of follow-the-leader principle. The step is quick and very short. The performers carry weapons and the leaders carry horns, which they blow at intervals. The performers are largely restricted in their behaviour, and are supposed to consume large quantities of meat, if available. They must drink no milk or beer and must abstain from sexual intercourse. This dance in Mwimbe was formerly always followed by a raid, in which all young warriors tried to find

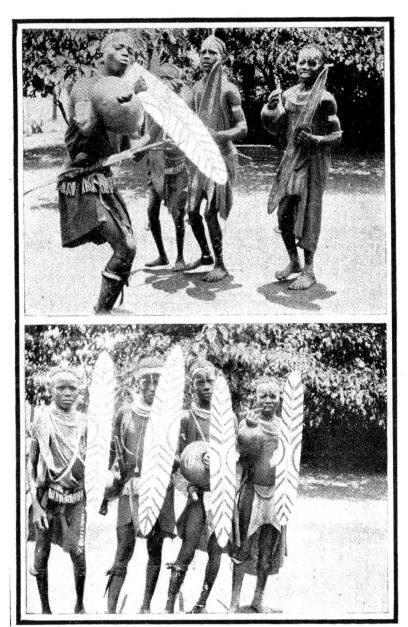

BROKEN GOURD DANCE.

Note the Warrior's sword worn on the right side and the dancing shieldin carried the left-hand ; also the white chalk patches round the eyes.

EMBU BOYS' PRE-INITIATION DANCE.

Note the gourd cut to let the hand pass through making it a sort of armlet. On this the wearer taps with a piece of stick held in the fingers in time with the step of the dance,

an opportunity for blooding their spears in some unfortunate victim.

At the urgent request of all the warriors of the Mwimbe an elaborate performance of this dance took place, with my permission, near the Government station of Chuka in 1913, on the strict understanding that goats only were to be the subsequent victims. This dance was naturally bound to disappear with the establishment of law and order.

A somewhat similar dance exists in Emberre—*i.e.* *Nyucho*—but it does not appear to be necessarily connected with war. It is danced after the millet is reaped, and the general rules governing it are much the same, though the dance is by no means so elaborately carried out, nor does the doctor supervise the building of the central hut.

A characteristic Mwimbe dance for women is the *Mwangu*. The performers draw up in two lines, and two or four of them dance up and down between the lines with a quick sidling step, clapping their hands in time to the song. This should really be danced in a special dried-grass skirt falling from the waist to the knees. This is worn only on festive occasions, and seems to be an object of much satisfaction to the wearer.

The Emberre Dances.—The Emberre do not dance as much as their neighbours. The dances which they do perform are, however, well executed and elaborate, while their singing is distinctly superior to that of the Kikuyu or the Embu.

Dances

The precircumcision dance for the boys (*Mguru*) resembles the *Mgiru* dance of the Embu, but is danced by boys only, and is highly elaborate. The performers paint their faces with a white circle all round, and characteristic patches about the eyes. This is to avert the ill luck which would otherwise follow their remarks or their glances. The body is also painted in fantastic patches, stripes of white ashes and charcoal forming the paint. Round the neck are worn strings of short lengths of grass and reeds strung as beads, and round the waist is worn a fringe of reeds, black seeds and cowrie shells. A flap of catskin is worn over the private parts, and a larger piece is worn over the right buttock. A head-dress of guinea-fowl and ostrich feathers is fixed on, and a bell is strapped to the right leg; on the right arm is carried a broken gourd as a wristlet. The fingers hold a little stick a few inches long, with which the gourd is tapped in time to the song, while in the left hand is carried the long dancing-shield of painted wood, or alternatively a lance seven to ten feet in length, tipped with long double streamers of string mounted with fur or grass-tufted at the ends. These lances are set up to mark the limits of the dancing-ground, and seem to have some effect in preventing harm resulting from the remarks made in the course of this song. The party is drawn up in two files, each faced by its leader. The dance consists of a monotonous stamping, scratching step, the performers sinking on the knees and rising again. A second figure consists of the same dance, with the performers arranged in a circle.

Dances

The song is extemporized, and consists of comments on people and incidents, frequently very personal and pointed. For instance, anyone who has not received the dancers hospitably is pilloried in their song, since the dancers go round among the neighbouring villages.

This dance is to be found in a much less elaborate form in Embu.

Steps.—Whatever the dance, the main feature is the step, rather than any other movement; many dances, indeed, entail no change of position, and the performers stand for hours on the same spot. In other cases a ring is formed in which one or two performers in turn take the principal part. These steps are very complicated, though often seemingly simple and easily copied; the rhythm, however, and the odd and unexpected interruptions are very strange to European spectators. As a rule the beat of the foot comes in the intervals of the tune, and not in time to it: the shuffle, scrape and hop which figure so frequently are also difficult to pick up.

Dances are fast growing common to all sections; the peculiar ones formerly to be found in limited areas are disappearing, while the more popular Kikuyu dances are spreading widely.

In some form or other, this exercise forms the main relaxation and social festivity of the native; it is very widely popular, and is practised by nearly all classes of the community. In Chuka, indeed, it is difficult to find a moment of day or night when the music and

Dances

drums of a dance cannot be heard somewhere in the distance. To European eyes many of the movements appear suggestive, if not actually indecent, but it seems doubtful if the native finds them so: certainly the dances do not appear to encourage immorality, though, of course, social gatherings which continue all night, under very free-and-easy conditions, can scarcely fail to permit opportunities for licence. It is as well to remember, however, that the Indian Mahommadan finds an English ballroom a most shocking sight; so it may well be that the European view of a native dance is unduly censorious. In any case, dances will almost certainly continue to feature largely in native life, and it is difficult to see how they could be replaced.

CHAPTER XVII

Diviners & Doctors

MAGIC plays a very large part in native life, and the slightest knowledge of the people is sufficient to bring one into contact with some form of superstition. The subject may be regarded as embracing all forms of the supernatural, from religious belief down to charms and amulets for daily wear.

The whole social life of the native is permeated by the rules of conduct summed up in the word *thahu* (ceremonial uncleanness). This may arise from a great variety of causes, some of them of a serious nature, such as homicide, others being, apparently, purely accidental, such as the collapsing of a house. A man who becomes for any of these many reasons *thahu* (unclean) must go through a more or less elaborate ceremony with a doctor, according to the degree of his uncleanness, the more serious cases involving the killing of a goat. Until this has been done he is unfit for general society and cannot associate with his fellows. This system is at once so well established, and yet so complicated, that it is very difficult for a European unacquainted with it to grasp the degree to which it influences the native mind. For instance, an excellent workman on a plantation becomes through some accident unclean, with the result that his employer is faced with a demand for a holiday of a day or two to enable the man to visit the native doctor. The request appears unreasonable and is refused, and the man is therefore compelled either to live as an outcast, shunned by his fellow-workmen, or else to run away from his employment. The situation upsets the whole gang, while at the same time they are probably quite unable to explain to their white employer what is worrying them. To them the situation appears to be as unpleasant and unreasonable as if they were asked to live with a man suffering from leprosy or smallpox. The employer, however, is probably quite unable to understand this view, and having satisfied himself that the man is not diseased, he cannot understand the general objection to him. Incidents such as this are frequently the cause of trouble among working gangs of the more primitive tribes.

This is the explanation of the dominating influence of the *mundu mugo*, or doctor. This functionary, in addition to his duties in connection with ceremonial uncleanness (for certain minor cases of uncleanness can be purged by any elder), also makes the numerous small charms which the average native likes to wear to guard him against sickness, wild animals, fatigue, etc. The doctor will also practise various ceremonies and sell small charms for curing ailments, or he may take to another branch of science and become a diviner.

Magic & Religion

In all such cases he may be regarded as comparatively harmless, and although he exists by preying upon the credulity of his neighbours, he is seldom responsible for a worse result than reluctance to consult a European doctor.

Ceremonial uncleanness may result from a number of causes, of which the following are the principal :—

1. Killing a human being, either in the more serious form of murder or in the lighter form of accident.[1]

2. Throwing out the dead, or touching a corpse.

3. A hyena leaving dung outside the hut.

4. The collapse of the hut, or the fall of a tree upon the subject.

5. The breaking of the marital bed, or a child getting upon it.

6. A woman stepping across her husband's legs.

7. Connection with a woman during her courses.

8. Killing a hyena; and, with certain sections, the killing of the " name animal " of the subject.

Also, generally, being cursed by an elder; or committing any act contrary to the " wisdom of the elders," such as eating prohibited food, or infringing one of the more important of the many social rules.

A far more sinister figure than the *mundu mugo* is the *mganga*, or witch-doctor, who practises black magic, or, in a less pernicious form, divination. This individual will sell curses and charms of great potency against enemies. He also professes to detect people who possess the evil eye, or who have the amiable habit of turning themselves into beasts of prey at night. He is frequently called in to explain such an incident as an epidemic, a drought or a bad harvest, when he is very apt to pitch upon some unfortunate old creature as the responsible person, with serious and possibly fatal results to his victim. These men are very greatly feared, and a clever and unscrupulous wizard of this type may sometimes wield a most undesirable influence. Nevertheless, occasionally, when they have reached the point of terrorizing the community, the tolerance of their neighbours breaks down, and concerted action is taken to put a stop to their ill doings by driving the offender away or even drowning him. These men must be regarded as a thoroughly evil influence. Since their powers depend upon the credulity and superstition of the people, they are bitterly opposed to progress and enlightenment in any direction, and are thus a frequent obstacle to good government. At an early stage of administration I was myself vigorously opposed by one of these men, who was eventually captured and imprisoned for his responsibility in the brutal ill treatment of an unfortunate old man. So furious was this wizard's old brother at this Government action that he lay in wait for my party on the march, and nothing but the prompt use of a revolver and the ready action of my police saved us from almost certain fatal results from the four poisoned arrows which he discharged at us before he was discovered and overcome.

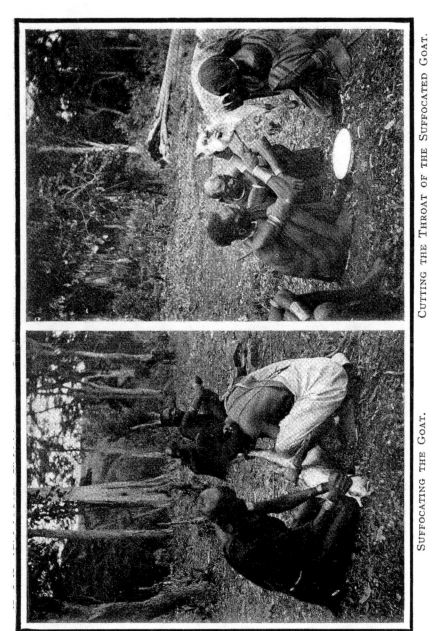

SUFFOCATING THE GOAT.

CUTTING THE THROAT OF THE SUFFOCATED GOAT.

Note the dish to catch the blood.

Magic & Religion

The office of doctor in either white or black magic does not seem to have been in any way hereditary, but was seemingly kept up by a sort of apprenticeship, the wizard instructing a likely young man, who in time succeeded to his magic gourds, bags, horns and other paraphernalia.

These men do not seem to have possessed any unusual powers or knowledge, and their great influence was presumably due to bluffing, combined with a shrewd use of such coincidences as could be twisted to support their pretensions. I have never personally seen any instance in which the remedies of the native doctor appeared to have any effect other than what can be readily explained as a species of faith healing.

Divination is an important branch of the doctor's art, and it forms the ready solution for any puzzling problem, such as the loss of property, outbreak of illness, etc.

The following is an account of an Embu *mganga's* procedure. The point to be enlightened was the loss of a white woollen scarf; this had disappeared, and some suspicion attached to a dismissed house-boy. The *mganga* was told that the scarf had disappeared, but was not told of any suspected person. He arrived with an assistant, and brought his skin bag, which contained about half-a-dozen gourds holding various " medicines " for different purposes; on the side of the bag was slung the hollow and charred shell of a small tortoise—a peculiarity of this *mganga's* bag. A straw mat was brought and spread for the operations;

and my representative (my gun-bearer) sat down at one side to ask the necessary questions, etc. Various other people sat near to assist in counting beads and so forth. The *mganga* then took out his large gourd from his bag, it being ovoid in shape, about ten inches long. Its narrow neck was stopped with a tuft of cow's tail, on which was wedged what seemed to be an old umbrella ring. In this gourd were some three hundred or more counters or beads: the great majority were black beans, but numerous other objects also appeared: several small stones, two or three pieces of wood, a bullet, a piece of amber pipe mouthpiece, and one or two other odds and ends. The *mganga* then took this gourd; the question as to the fate of the scarf was asked by the questioner, who then made a sort of repeated spitting motion with the tongue and lips. The *mganga* then took the gourd, waved it in the air, repeated the slight spitting, took out the stopper and emptied out some counters; of these he made a heap, shaking out a small handful several times; he then made two more heaps, about the same size —*i.e.* containing some sixty or eighty counters. The number of handfuls tipped out of the gourd for each heap seemed quite optional. The three heaps stood for (1) theft, (2) loss, (3) mislaying. The counters were then counted in tens and twenties, and the result told to the *mganga*. After a moment's thought he stated that the scarf was neither lost nor definitely stolen, but that it had been washed and put out to dry, and that someone had taken a fancy to it. Apparently

" theft " would only have been the taking of the scarf from its own proper place (his house). This completed the first stage. Now to identify the man who took the scarf.

It was considered that one of five people must be the culprit, so the spectators chose five sticks, one to represent each possible thief. These were carefully identified and given to the *mganga*, who was unaware whom they represented. He then produced a small gourd with some chalk or similar substance in it. This he tipped into his left palm; he then took up the five sticks—the originals of which he did not know—and chalked their ends. He then licked up some of the chalk, and rubbed some on his forehead. He then had the question put, as before, with the spitting; he held up the sticks, murmured some words—in which the scarf was mentioned—waved the sticks round his head, arranged them side by side in his hand, and pressed them firmly against his forehead. There they stuck for a moment, falling down one after the other; two fell almost together, after the other three. These were carefully noted. All the five sticks were then arranged in a circle, chalked ends inwards; piles of counters were tipped out for each, and counted; the result of this was to indicate one of the two sticks which fell last as belonging to the culprit; but which one was unknown. Five more sticks were chosen, therefore, and the ceremony was repeated. This time also, two sticks were indicated, but only one of them represented one of the two men selected by the previous choice. Therefore the man who was indicated each time was the culprit. This man was the discharged house-boy, the result being received as a striking example of the success of the system.

It may be remarked that the result was the expected one; but the *mganga* certainly did not know which stick represented the suspected boy, and it was either a curious coincidence or else a very neat piece of trickery—too neat for Embu natives; unless the claim to powers of divination is to be believed. It was unfortunately impossible to prove the guilt or innocence of the supposed culprit. No special ceremony concluded the performance, and no great reverence or respect was shown by the spectators, though they evidently firmly believed in the proceedings.

This system seems to be the same with most sections; in the above case the onlookers were Nyeri Kikuyu, Ndia Kikuyu, Embu and Chuka, all of whom seemed quite satisfied with the procedure.

In addition to divination, the *mganga*, as well as the *mundu mugo*, acts as a doctor for the cure of diseases, and is called in, just as his European confrère, when anyone is at all seriously ill. The proceedings are of a magical nature, and the underlying idea appears to be purification, or the casting out of the cause of the disease, rather than the administration of any remedies which might have a physical effect.

The actual ceremony performed depends upon the case in question, and on the methods of the old man who carries out the cure; but the general principles remain the same, and the different practitioners vary from each other only in detail. As a rule when a person falls ill a search is made for some cause of the trouble; this generally affords some old man an opportunity to remind the relatives that he at some remote date performed a ceremony for that particular person, with a view to protecting him from illness, but that the conditions at that time contemplated have in some way been altered; hence the illness. This is an excellent reason for employing the same old man to carry out a cure, and as in most cases the disease is of a temporary nature, it is to be expected that the patient will recover sooner or later, which is duly credited to the powers of the doctor. Failing some ostensible and obvious reason, recourse must be had to the general explanation that someone who has a grudge against the victim has bewitched him, in which case the same remedy is needed, so that under all circumstances the faculty profit very satisfactorily.

The following is given as a good example of the methods generally employed.

The case was that of a girl who had come to live in the Government station with an Embu native (my servant) residing there. Some months later she contracted a severe cold and fever, consequent upon living in a hut with a leaky roof. I gave her quinine and suitable medicines, but the cure took longer than was considered reasonable, and search was made for the cause for a protracted illness. This was at once forthcoming from an old man, who recalled the fact that he had some years previously carried out a ceremony which was to ensure the good health of the girl as long as she remained in the village; since she had now gone to live elsewhere, she had, of course, become ill. He therefore attended with all the necessary paraphernalia to effect a cure.

In a suitable open spot near the hut of the sick girl he placed a flat stone; he then found some grass, which he cut up small with a little knife, leaving the resultant mince on the stone. He then produced from his bags two horns, apparently bush-buck horns cut down; these were stood up on end on either side of the stone. A small fire of twigs was made, and a gourd was put ready near the horns.

The husband of the girl then produced a he-goat, which was thrown down and partially suffocated by holding the windpipe and nostrils; when nearly dead, the animal was revived by the old man, who stroked it down the head and back and put snuff into its nostrils, muttering invocations to it to recover as he did so. He then took it up by the legs and swung it round the little fire, muttering at the same time some words which appeared to be commands to the disease to depart; this was done as he stood facing the hut. The unfortunate goat was again held down by the old man and his assistant, and finally suffocated. The doctor then muttered some words to the effect that the goat would absorb the disease; a friend of the husband then held the animal upside down on his shoulder, with the head hanging down in front of his chest.

The doctor's assistant then stabbed the animal in the throat and the blood which gushed out was caught in a pan put underneath; the two horns and the gourd were also held under the dripping blood, and four small brushes also received a few drops, these little brushes having been previously made from bunches of grass tied round the stem. (Certain grasses are apparently desirable for this purpose, but they do not seem to be particularly uncommon or remarkable, nor are they always the same; it seems probable that each practitioner uses his own prescription, which he varies to suit his convenience.)

The goat is then cut up and skinned in the usual way, beginning at the throat; the joints are severed, and the various organs are taken out. This is done on banana leaves spread on the ground.

Three dishes are then prepared, containing powdered charcoal, blood from the goat, and water in which is the grass previously cut up. These are placed near the stone, and the lungs and heart of the goat are tied to the doctor's bags, which are then swung round the stone and the other objects, a piece of gut serving to secure the bags together. The lungs are then detached from the bags, and the doctor blows them out, exhausting them again into each of the dishes in turn.

The sick girl now arrives, and is seated on a mat facing the stone. The husband is seated next to her, and a piece of creeper is placed across their feet (the variety of creeper is immaterial). A tuft of grass is picked and placed between the girl's toes.

The doctor then takes the lungs again, and inflates them, exhausting them into the girl's mouth and ears, murmuring a charm as he does so. The grass brushes are then brought, and the doctor throws blood over her head with them; an oryx horn is produced from one of the bags, and the assistant puts the base of this on her head, mutters a few words, and waves it round her.

The doctor then comes with the two horns and his ceremonial wooden spoon, all marked down the centre with a chalk line. These are held by him, together with a foot of the goat, in front of her; he draws them down her body from her face, and commands the disease to go to Kirinyagga (Mount Kenya); he then switches her and the husband in the face with the grass brushes. The assistant then holds the goat's foot to her head, shoulders and breasts. The husband puts his arm in hers, and the horns and foot are again drawn down her; the husband and his friend then take the horns and the foot and hold them across the girl, in front of her. The doctor takes the brushes and draws them down the girl again, and dips them into the three dishes in turn; they are then thrust into the husband's mouth, and afterwards the girl's, each of whom spits after each application of the brush. The assistant next comes and does the drawing action from behind the husband, and subsequently from under the husband's legs as he sits on the ground. The lungs are again brought and blown out, the doctor exhausting them through the brushes into the girl's face; the horns and brushes are waved about, while the

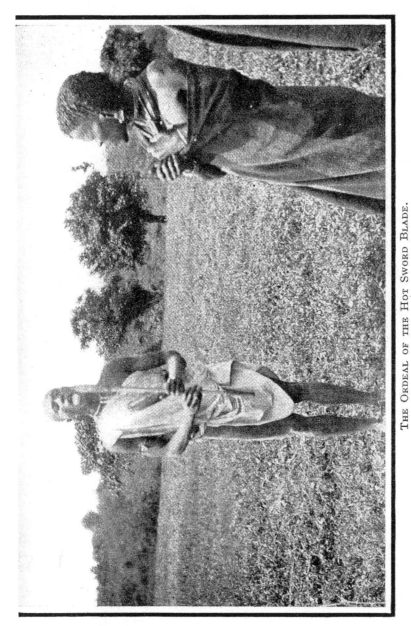

THE ORDEAL OF THE HOT SWORD BLADE.

The sword blade is heated to just below red heat, and three chalk marks are smeared across it, and the witness has to lick these off.

doctor murmurs an incantation. He then gives the girl a horn to drink, containing water and blood; he unties the brushes, and dips them in blood and charcoal, with which he wipes the feet of the husband and the girl. The latter stands up, and the doctor brushes her down the whole length of the body with the blood and charcoal. She is then helped back to her hut, while the assistant follows her behind, brushing the backs of her feet with the blood and charcoal. The meat has meanwhile been cooked on the little fire, and this is eaten by the doctor and his assistant, and one or two old men who have come as spectators; the remains of the animal are carefully carried off into the woods and thrown away. The various properties are packed up, and the ceremony is at an end.

The girl wears the skin of the goat round her waist, as a garment, as soon as it can be cleaned; this is considered to complete the cure.

The whole ceremony is very elaborate, and to a civilized onlooker disgusting; but it must be remembered that the effect on the mind of the patient is very great, and therefore helps materially to effect a cure. Indeed, were the sufferer restricted to the remedies of civilization, and prevented from carrying out the native practice, it is more than probable that he—or even more she—would remain very ill, or even die, from mental depression and fear; but it is singularly annoying to see really efficacious European remedies abandoned in favour of such methods.

In the above instance the girl recovered rapidly,

probably owing to the fact that she was already well on the way to convalescence, but also, no doubt, partly owing to the mental effect of the ceremony. It was quite clear to me, however, that the case was regarded as a striking illustration of the triumph of native methods over European, though naturally no one actually expressed that view to me. It is probably not so much that the native disbelieves the efficacy of European medicine, but that he mistrusts any proceedings which do not include some sort of magic. Were the European to include some kind of mystic ceremony in his treatment, it is probable that he would make a far greater impression and effect many more cures than he can as long as he restricts himself to honest methods.

Curiously enough, the argument, " Physician, heal thyself," does not seem to appeal to the native mind at all. On the occasion described above, the doctor was suffering from an advanced stage of elephantiasis in both feet; he explained that he was unable to perform upon himself, and that any rival would probably merely make him worse, out of jealousy!

The incantations used were hard to obtain; the doctor refused to repeat them, and they were said so fast, in such a mumbling manner, that it was very hard for any bystander to follow what was mentioned. It seems very doubtful, however, if any set formula is used; occasionally a Swahili word will be detected, and references are made to bystanders or the particular case; probably the general sense of the remarks

Magic & Religion

is unaltered, but the doctor composes the actual form as he goes along. No reference to a deity seems to be made, except in a very vague sort of way; there is nothing like an actual prayer, nor is the attention of the doctor directed to any particular quarter. Mount Kenya is frequently referred to, but for no special reason, apparently. Very little can be obtained in the way of explanation or reason for what is done, and this seems to be not so much from reluctance on the part of the doctor as sheer inability.

Such ceremonies can be witnessed by anyone interested, no class being excluded; strangers are regarded with some suspicion, but anyone known to be friendly is quite welcome.

NOTE

[1] Compare the case of the Phrygian who came to Sardis to implore Crœsus to purify him from the stain of blood according to the customs of the country (Herodotus, Book I., chapter 35).

CHAPTER XVIII

MAGIC & RELIGION (*continued*)

Oaths & Ordeals

THE numerous disputes which are brought before the Elders' Councils give rise to endless opportunities for the use of oaths and ordeals. As a rule each witness will give his evidence without any preamble or affirmation, but in more serious cases where there is only the witnesses' word to rely upon, or when the evidence is conflicting, an oath or a trial by ordeal is often resorted to by the puzzled old men. This has frequently an astonishing effect, and I have often seen cases where one or other party refused to take the prescribed oath, preferring to lose the case. This view, however, is restricted to the more primitive savages, sophisticated young men being often quite cynical over the taking of an oath.

The stone, or other object, with holes in it, used for ordeals by the Akikuyu and Akamba, and preserved by a special custodian, does not appear among the Embu tribes; they know of such things, however, and would probably treat one with considerable respect and apprehension were they asked to take part in a ceremony including the use of one.

Trial by Ordeal. The Heated Knife.—This is the

popular method of disposing of a disputed case, when there are numerous witnesses on either side who swear to entirely contrary facts (a very ordinary occurrence). The ordeal consists in licking a hot sword blade. The *Kiama* (Elders' Council) assembles with the interested parties, and in the centre is made a small fire of hot ashes. A *mundu mugo* (doctor) is called, and he brings with him his medicine gourd. He heats a sword in the fire until it is just below red heat. Across the blade he smears three bars of white paste, made of ash, about half-an-inch wide, and the same distance apart. The sword being at the right heat (cauterizing, but not red, heat), he hands it to the first of the two disputants. This man has to lick the blade so as to remove some of the paste from all three of the bars. The sword is then reheated, and the second party licks it in the same manner; if necessary, witnesses are also called upon to lick the sword. Those who have undergone the ordeal then walk slowly round the circle, showing their tongues; the one whose tongue is most blistered is considered to be telling lies. This ordeal often results in a true verdict, owing to the party in the wrong fearing the result and refusing to undergo the trial. If, however, the ordeal is undertaken, it usually results in both parties being more or less severely burnt, when the Elders conclude that " both are lying " and dismiss the case, having eaten the goat or goats paid as " Court Fees." Other forms of ordeal exist, but this is the most popular, to which almost any disputant will appeal in case of doubt.

Magic & Religion

It should be noted that it is quite possible to perform this test by proxy; and people are surprisingly willing to undergo the ordeal for a friend or acquaintance, even when they can have little knowledge of the rights of the case.

Naturally, also, the method lends itself to all sorts of ingenious trickery, and dodges to circumvent the effect of the hot iron; so much so that a man will sometimes boast in confidence that he can always defeat an opponent at this form of ordeal.

As an alternative to a test such as the above, a solemn oath is sometimes administered, which is supposed to extort the truth by the serious character of the supernatural results expected to overtake any offender against its sanctity.

The " Ngondu " Oath.—The following is an account of the oath to which great respect is paid by all sections. The ceremony is to be found among all the tribes, though it differs in details. The Embu method is as follows.

A small goat is brought, and its head is tied with a rope so as to prevent it moving. It is then, while alive, flayed from the neck to half-way down the back, the skin being slit over the backbone and turned back for several inches; the eyes are blinded by having four thorns thrust through them. The miserable animal is left in this condition, standing in the middle of the group, while the first man to swear the oath declaims the facts to which he is swearing. He then comes forward and plunges his spear into the animal's ribs, murmuring at the same time that he wishes he may die if he has not spoken the truth. His rival then comes up and does the same thing. The goat falls dead and is carried off and burnt whole; should any part of it be eaten, it would produce serious illness. The effect of this oath is that the perjured party dies in a year or less.

The main difference among the sections is that the Embu and the Chuka use a spear to kill the animal, while the Ndia Kikuyu, the Emberre and the Mwimbe use a club to dispatch the beast.

This oath is supposed to be an exceptionally solemn one, and all the natives profess great fear of it; this, however, does not eliminate cases of what is to a European incontrovertible perjury; it is quite possible that these cases are not so in the eyes of the natives, in spite of this fact, since the native idea of truth is so odd that two parties will flatly contradict each other over some detail of fact, each believing his story to be perfectly true. It is not very frequently resorted to: I witnessed the ceremony only once, though this was chiefly owing to my dislike of the treatment accorded to the wretched goat. This is a curious example of the callousness of the native; while far from naturally cruel, he considers the feelings of an animal little more than we should sympathize with a peeled potato.

The Chuka perform a somewhat similar ceremony to add solemnity to the findings of the Elders' Council: the following is a description of a typical case.

The dispute was over a runaway wife, who preferred

the defendant to her rightful husband, the plaintiff;
the latter therefore brought an action to ask the aid
of the Council either to secure the return of his wife,
or to carry out a divorce according to native law, by
the payment of the original dowry by the defendant to the plaintiff. The woman and the defendant,
however, stoutly maintained that the husband had ill-
treated his wife, who was therefore perfectly justified
in deserting him without further formality. Since
the evidence resolved itself into the narration of
conflicting statements, the Elders had recourse to an
oath.

Each party produced a goat, and these animals were
then killed by being speared by two of the Elders;
they were then skinned (a diamond-shaped piece being
left on the breast of each), and selected scraps of the
meat were made up into little parcels in banana leaf.
The defendant then stood on the blood-stained leaves
on which the goats had been killed, and related his
story; as he did so, he held in his hand one of the
banana-leaf packets of scraps, from which he ate the
raw scraps at intervals, beginning by throwing one
over his head. The Elders were meanwhile uttering
curses on perjury, and listening to his statement.
The plaintiff followed with his statement under similar
conditions, and the Elders considered their verdict.
They announced, however, that the case was too difficult for them to settle, so, at the suggestion of a chief
who was standing by, but taking no actual part, the
Elders decided to leave the matter to be settled by

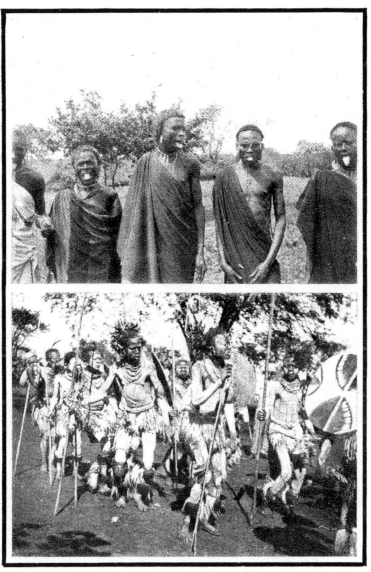

ORDEAL OF THE HOT SWORD BLADE.

Showing the tongues after licking the hot sword to determine which witness has
burnt his tongue owing to having told lies in evidence.

EMBU BOYS' PRE-INITIATION DANCE.

Note the shield worn on the left arm by means of a block left projecting from
the wood of the shield through which the arm is thrust.

the virtue of their magical powers. They clapped their hands, and pronounced a curse which would prove fatal to the perjurer within a year; the two diamond-shaped pieces of goatskin were made into rings for each party to wear, under pain of the extreme penalty of the oath, the survivor being obviously in the right.

As a matter of fact, in this case, both parties survived; the woman continued to live with the defendant, and the plaintiff allowed the matter to drop. I am inclined to believe that there was probably good ground for the accusation of ill-treatment. Anyhow, the oath appeared to serve its purpose fairly well, and did no particular harm. It is obvious, however, that such methods must fall into disrepute as the native becomes more civilized, while it is of course impossible to admit such a ritual into judicial proceedings under European auspices.

There is another curious branch of magic, which deals with the control of Nature: rain, drought, insects, etc., are supposed to be influenced by the incantation of certain doctors. This power also often goes with certain clans or professions; for instance, among the Ndia Kikuyu, the Ithaga clan (who are mostly smiths) are supposed to be the masters of specially potent curses, and to be able to ward off or summon rain: I know of several cases where general indignation was caused by the alleged action of a smith in preventing rain for a considerable period. The localized bursts of rain which are one of the characteristics of this mountainous region are probably largely responsible for this idea.

A doctor is often employed against insect pests also. I remember one very successful incantation which freed the country-side from a serious plague of caterpillars! This was considered a most creditable performance. A cynical observer, however, might have taken the view that the old gentleman was cautious enough to avoid action until he knew from previous observation that the plague was reaching the stage where it would disappear from natural causes.

Such ideas die hard, and any coincidence is seized upon to bolster them up: in most cases, however, they do not do much harm, beyond enabling some old scamp to live comfortably on his neighbours' credulity. Can no similar instance be found in European society? Occasionally some such doctor, however, may obtain an undesirable amount of power, but I found in practice that it was not difficult to weaken this, by challenging him to do something which he knew very well he could not hope to achieve, such as the wiping out of a plague of locusts on their first appearance, or the prompt production of rain in a settled drought. The difficulty was sufficient to make him admit impotence, with corresponding effect on the hearers.

The Evil Eye.—There is a widespread belief in the power of the evil eye, or something akin to it; numerous persons are supposed to have the power of causing a definite harmful effect to people or animals merely by looking at them; in particular, they must on no account praise the object. This faculty may be accidental, in which case it is regarded as a personal misfortune, or it may be acquired by a wizard and definitely used by him for his own ends. The *mundu mugo*, or beneficent doctor, generally sells small charms —usually little pieces of wood to be worn on a string round the neck or wrist—which are supposed to protect the wearer from the ill effects of the evil eye.

The same idea appears also in other forms; words which are not meant really seriously may possibly acquire a dangerous potency, and become an effectual curse. Parents who abuse their children, even if it is done only in a fit of momentary irritation, may well find that they have brought misfortune on the child, when a doctor must be called in to purge the offence.

An instance of this accidental and unintentional " ill-wishing " is found in the pre-initiation dance of the boys, particularly in its Emberre form. During the dance a song is kept up in which friends or neighbours are freely criticized, but this is intended only as a joke, and no real harm is meant; nevertheless, damage might be done were no precautions taken. The performers therefore paint black rings round each eye, and a white line round the face and across the forehead; this neutralizes any ill effect that might ensue from glance or word. Why the danger arises in the first place, and why this painting removes it, the people seem unable to explain.

This attribute is not necessarily confined to natives ; I found that I was myself believed to have the power of pronouncing a sort of unintentional curse—that is to say, if I warned a man against something, it became very likely that that misfortune would overtake him. For instance, if I cautioned a messenger to beware of lions on some journey he became convinced that he would be taken by them, and would not set out until he had gone to a doctor for a counter-charm. The idea was a most inconvenient and annoying one, for it was impossible for me to caution a servant about carrying, say, a pile of plates carefully without being considered responsible for the smash which usually followed. In one instance my joking comparison of an extremely voluble and raucous-voiced old man with a hyena was construed into a threat to turn the old gentle-man actually into a hyena, a lot of explanation being necessary to convince all concerned that there was no danger of such a transformation. I know also of a case where a white man was believed to bring eventual disaster upon any native who worked for him ; it was generally admitted that he was quite a good and con-siderate employer, but he was unfortunately afflicted with this curious influence. So firmly rooted was the belief that I had the greatest difficulty in persuading a few natives to act even as porters to carry his loads for him.

There seems to be no explanation of the origin of

such attributes; they may occur in anyone, and are only found out by observation; there is no cure, and the effect can only be warded off by suitable charms.

The question of magic leads up to its foundation —religion; for all the claims of the doctors and the elders are based on alleged Divine authority, the theory being that the doctor understands more of the working of Divine laws than his neighbours, and that he is, in consequence, able to direct the working of those laws to some extent.

In common with the Kikuyu and the Meru, the Embu tribes have very little definite religion. A vague belief in a Creator certainly exists, and the snowy cap of Mount Kenya appears to be generally regarded as his residence; a wizard in the course of his incantations will implore Divine approval by addressing the mountain. There seems, however, to be very little idea of any definite Divine control of everyday life. Belief, in fact, would appear to be limited to the existence of a First Cause. Beyond this, Divine approval or displeasure functions only automatically through the working of social laws of uncleanness, purification, and so on. The name universally used for the Deity is the Masai word *Engai*. Sacred groves exist and are regarded with considerable respect, no trees being felled and no one living within them; I cannot, however, give any account from personal observation of any ceremony of a religious nature in one of these groves. There appears to be no idea of a future life, and it seems to be generally believed that a man once dead is completely finished. The theological system, there-fore, may be described as a vague theism, which forms the foundation and the authority for the elabo-rate system for the prohibitions and observances as expounded by the witch-doctors.[1]

All sections take readily to novel religious teaching. Both Christianity and Islam easily gain adherents. It is very doubtful, however, whether the new religion is taken seriously in the great majority of cases. Most natives will join readily in any novel religious cere-mony, the more spectacular the better; while an additional attraction exists in the shape of increased social prestige resulting from friendship and approval of the European or coast Swahili who is propagating the religion in question. It is not uncommon to see a nominal Christian native returning from a church service to arrange a marriage with a third or fourth wife, while a nominal convert to Islam has only too often no scruple about getting drunk. In fact, they appear to regard their new religion merely as a fashion or species of magic which need not be taken seriously as a controlling factor in everyday conduct.[2]

It is most unfortunate that the native who once loses his own primitive beliefs and superstitions ap-pears very rarely to find anything to take their place. Consequently there is a type which is only too com-mon, where original tribal discipline and belief have broken down, leaving the man devoid of any rules of conduct, thereby making him an easy prey to the more sophisticated vices of civilization.

Magic & Religion

NOTES

[1] "His religion has been made for him by others, communicated to him by tradition, determined to fixed forms by imitation, and retained by habit" (a singularly applicable description from *The Varieties of Religious Experience*, by William James).

[2] " The quarrels and divisions about religion were evils unknown to the heathen. The reason was, because the religion of the heathen consisted rather in rites and ceremonies than in any constant belief" (Bacon, Essay III.).

CHAPTER XIX

ON the whole, tradition is singularly neglected among the Embu tribes; old men have a hazy idea of the history of their fathers' times, but even that is unreliable and contradictory. No sort of tribal story is preserved, and it seems as if the natives were well content to accept things as they find them, without worrying about the past. Such records as are to be secured will be found incorporated in the chapters on History.

Genealogies are also scanty and unreliable: this perhaps is hardly to be wondered at, since little actual importance attaches to them, and the essentially practical outlook of the native, therefore, discards them as useless knowledge of no interest.

Folk-stories, however, exist among all sections, and are very apt to take a form similar to the nursery stories of Europe. There is usually no obvious moral and no perceptible original significance to the story. The plot tends to be alarming or gruesome, and usually has a considerable element of the supernatural. There is frequently a character of magical powers and attributes who is dangerous and alarming, usually with cannibalistic tendencies, but who has at

208

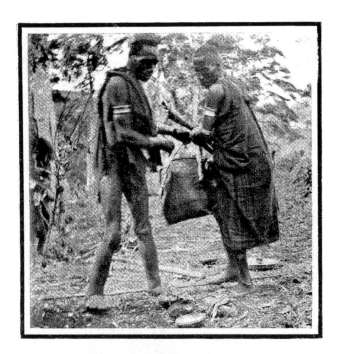

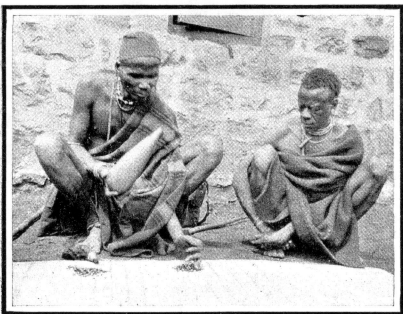

SWINGING THE DOCTOR'S BAG.

The bag and horns are swung round the dish of blood and other medicines.

EMBU DIVINER.

The Diviner is pouring out the seeds, pebbles, etc., with which his magic gourd is filled. These are piled in heaps, and he counts the numbers in each heap to arrive at his conclusions.

the same time a slightly comic aspect, being easily out-witted and defeated by a shrewd hero. This personage is perhaps best translated by the English word bogey, as it is used in the ordinary European nurses' stories; it may be either male or female, and seems to have no suggestion of any human origin, so that "ghost" would be quite a misleading term.

The best narrators are generally the old women, though it is often difficult to persuade them to display their powers. Once started on a story, however, they tell it really well, with a wealth of descriptive detail and pantomime. The voices of the various actors are carefully imitated, and a considerable amount of dramatic gesture gives life to the narrative, the crucial point of the story being usually emphasized by a most impressive howl, shriek or jump. In fact, for a childish audience it would be difficult to improve on one of these old ladies as a story-teller.

A selection of the stories follow, which vary in coherence and continuity. While as a rule they are quite well constructed as to plot and incident, some will be found which seem pointless, incoherent and brief. I have, therefore, given specimens of each type.

The Story of Kimangara.—Once upon a time a man named Kimangara went to buy a wife; and he also built a house for her to live in. Then when he brought the wife home, he said: "See, wife, I have no brothers; you must never ask me where they are." So the wife promised to remember this; but later on, when they had children, who grew up, the wife said: "Our children are big, it is high time that we had them circumcised; where is your brother, that he may attend the ceremony?" Then Kimangara said: "I told you never to ask me that question. Now make plenty of gruel." This they did, and they put it in some gourds. Then Kimangara went in search of his brethren; and he found many people who were brothers of his, but they all had wings. He invited them all to his village, and a very large number came. Then he asked his wife: "What can they eat?" And the wife said: "They must just share a gourd of gruel among them all." But Kimangara asked his wife: "What can they eat on the way home?" And his wife said: "Give them a second gourd of gruel to share. It seems to me that I have married a husband who can do nothing but walk about." But the brethren finished all the gruel, and a third gourd also, and Kimangara asked his wife once more: "What can they eat?" And the wife said: "You must give them a goat." And Kimangara did so, and the goat was eaten. And a second goat was given to them, and a third after that. And Kimangara said to his wife: "What shall I give them to eat?" And she said: "Give them one of our bullocks." And he did so, and they ate it; and two more bullocks after that. Then Kimangara said to his wife: "What shall I give them to eat?" And she said: "Give them the name of your father" (*i.e.* his eldest child). And he did so, and the brethren ate it. And he asked again, and his wife said: "Give them your mother's name" (*i.e.* his eldest daughter). And he did so, and the brethren ate her. And this they did until all the children were finished. Then the wife said: "Now you must give me to them." So Kimangara did so, and she was eaten. Then Kimangara saw that there was no one and nothing left to give to his brethren, so he grew very much afraid. He went into the hut, and he dug a pit, and he covered it with wood; then he hid himself inside. But a chameleon sitting at the top of the wall saw him. Then all the brethren, with their arms like birds' wings, came in, and they looked for Kimangara; but they would not have found him if the chameleon had not told them to look in the floor. Then they took away the earth that covered the hole, and Kimangara was hidden, all except his teeth; and by these one of the brethren drew him out of the hole. And they all ate him; and that was the end of Kimangara.

What the Bogey told the Children.—Once upon a time a Bogey went to look for children to eat. He found a party of them sitting together, and he asked them: "Where is your father?" So they replied: "He has gone to make spears." And the Bogey asked: "What for?" And they replied: "To kill bogeys." Then he said: "And where is Mutua?" And they replied: "He has gone to make spears to kill bogeys who eat children." Then the children asked the Bogey: "When a bogey eats children, what sort of meat are they like to eat?" And the Bogey answered: "They are like heart, like bird." And then he went away.

The Goat and the Kids and the Bogey.—A goat once went to a pit and produced a family, but a

Bogey saw her. And she had four children: the first was named "Kathengi Matumu"; the second was "Mathangu"; the third was "Kakomonge," and the fourth was "Mwenda Kuongo." And the goat called her children to give them milk, and she said: "Beware, there is a Bogey behind the house." Then she went out, and the Bogey came and called the kids in a deep voice. But they knew that the voice was not their mother's, and they only jeered at the Bogey. And this happened three times.

So the Bogey went to a wizard for assistance, and the wizard said: "You must go to the *siafu* [biting ant] to get your tongue shaved down, and then your voice will sound like the mother goat's." So the Bogey did this, though the ants hurt most terribly, and it was only possible to get a small piece of the tongue cut down each day. But at last the tongue was small enough, and the Bogey went and called to the children of the goat. So the kids all came out, and the Bogey ate three of them, but the eldest, "Kathengi Matumu," asked to be spared, saying that he would be a slave to the Bogey if he were spared. So she spared him, and took him home to her house. Soon after this the Bogey had a child, and when the child was big enough it went with Kathengi Matumu to watch the crops, to prevent all the wild animals from eating them. Then one day Kathengi Matumu took a spear and sharpened it, and stabbed a baobab-tree, and said: "When this tree dies the eater of my brothers will die." But the child of the Bogey grew angry, and threatened to tell its mother. But Kathengi Matumu said: "I was only in fun." However, the next day the same thing took place, and this time the Bogey's child told its mother. But the mother asked Kathengi Matumu, and he said: "It was only a charm to kill all the animals that come to eat the crops." But the next day the tree fell down, and Kathengi Matumu killed the Bogey's child, and skinned it. He took the meat to the Bogey, and said: "This is the meat of one of the animals that eat your crops, and your child has stopped behind to watch the skin, which is put out to dry." Then Kathengi Matumu sharpened a spear; and the Bogey said: "Where is my child?" And he said: "Only just behind." But the Bogey asked again, so Kathengi Matumu said: "How can you ask, when you know that you ate it!" But the Bogey was very angry when the truth was told, and said to Kathengi Matumu: "I shall kill you as soon as I have sharpened my razor." But when the razor was sharp, Kathengi Matumu did not wait to be attacked, but stabbed the Bogey with his spear. But he heard a voice inside from his eldest brother, which said, "Don't kill me," and the brother came out. Then Kathengi Matumu stabbed again, and his second brother was recovered in the same way, and the Bogey died. Then they all went home to their mother, who had remained living in the same place all the time. They called at the door, but their mother refused to believe them at first, saying: "How can you be my children, even if you have their voices, since my children were all eaten by the Bogey?" But at last she believed them, and they went into the house, and they all lived happily together after that, having been shaved on their return home.

In addition to stories of the kind related above, there are also numerous nature stories, which give explanations of the habits of animals, natural phenomena, and so forth. These are not regarded as stories meant only for children (as the folk-tales above related are), but are frequently quoted by anyone as explanations of physical facts. It is somewhat doubtful whether the average native really believes them: rather, perhaps, he knows them and accepts them in lieu of anything better: his attitude is somewhat agnostic in this as in other matters, and he regards such accounts as being worthy of note, perhaps, but not admitting of investigation, and, above all, without effect on practical details of daily life.

The following stories were both obtained from men round the camp-fire, and are fairly typical of their kind.

The Elephant and the Chameleon.—The Elephant is afraid of the Chameleon for the following reason. Once upon a time the Chameleon met the Elephant in the forest, and the Elephant said to the Chameleon: "Why is it that you walk like me, and swing and hesitate over each step? You are not strong and heavy like me, and there can be no need for you to examine the ground before you walk on it, as I have to do." The Chameleon replied: "On the contrary,

I am even larger and stronger than you, although it suits me to disguise the fact." The Elephant could not believe this, and he challenged the Chameleon to prove the truth of his words. So the Chameleon arranged that they should meet the next day and the Elephant should be convinced of the truth of the Chameleon's statement.

The Chameleon then went to the place where the meeting had been arranged, and dug a large hole, which he roofed very carefully with sticks and grass, so that it looked like the rest of the ground and yet would give way beneath the slightest weight.

Then he waited for the Elephant's arrival, and when the latter came, the Chameleon asked him if he could stamp on the ground with such force that he would bury himself in the pit which would result. The Elephant said that he certainly could do no such thing, and asked if the Chameleon could. To this the Chameleon replied that he would have no difficulty at all in doing so, and with that he jumped into the air, alighting on the prepared pit. The covering gave way and the Chameleon disappeared from sight. The Elephant was so much alarmed by this exhibition of power on the part of an animal that appeared so weak that he rushed away in great haste, so much so that he broke one tusk in his flight.

Now the Elephant warns all the other beasts not to trust the Chameleon, who is the most powerful beast of any, though he does not look like it. That is the reason why the Elephant fears the Chameleon to this day.

Why the Mole fears the Sun.—Very long ago the Sun made some medicine that should raise all dead people to life again; they would only need to have some put on their lips when they died and they would at once rise up again.

Having made this medicine, the Sun chose as his messenger the Mole, which was, at that time, a beast that ran about on the surface of the ground. The Sun gave the packet containing the medicine to the Mole, with instructions to carry it to all men; so the Mole set out on his journey.

On the way he met the Hyena, who stopped him to ask on what message he was going. So the Mole told him about the new medicine which had been made by the Sun, and showed the parcel of it.

The Hyena was much upset by this news—" For," said he, " what am I to eat, if there are no more nice fresh corpses for me to live on? You, Mole, have always been a friend of mine, so do me one favour; take this packet of medicine from me, and give me the packet that the Sun gave to you." Now the medicine of the Hyena was meant to kill all men, so that there would be many corpses.

The Mole was somewhat uneasy about this, but he wished to oblige an old friend, so he gave up the packet of medicine that had come from the Sun, and took that of the Hyena instead, and the Hyena went off well satisfied.

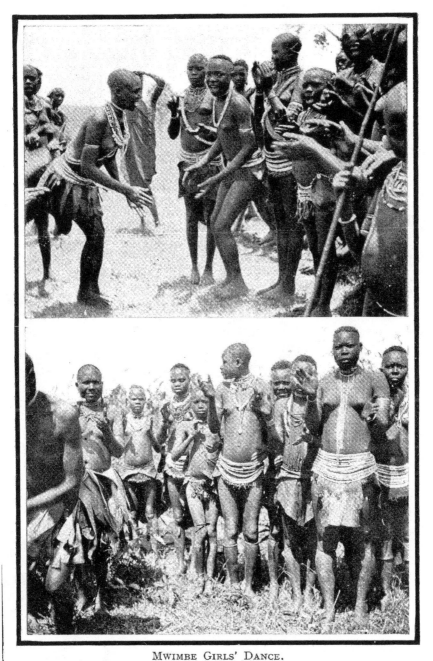

MWIMBE GIRLS' DANCE.

The dance consists of a side step rapidly opposite a partner, both clapping hands.

MWIMBE WOMEN'S DANCE.

The old women take the active part while the girls stand in a line and clap.

But the mole was uneasy about the affair, so he returned to the Sun, and told him all that had happened, and showed the medicine which the Hyena had given him. The Sun was very angry, and said: " You have lost the medicine which I had made with so much trouble, and now I cannot make any more ; I trusted you to take my message, and you have failed ; henceforth you shall fear my face, and hide when you see me." The Mole went away much ashamed, and since that time he has lived beneath the earth ; if he sees the face of the Sun he dies. The Hyena was not punished, since he was only looking after his own interests ; he and Mankind hated each other long before that. But if the Hyena's medicine had reached Mankind, all people would have died. As it is, they are neither better nor worse off than they were before the Sun made the medicine.

In addition to stories to explain natural features, there are various explanations offered which are merely attempts to account for the facts of nature. The following are specimens of these.

Sun.—The Mwimbe say that the sun is sent out from the house of Mukuna Ruko, whose body is all eyes. There are many bridges leading to this house far away in the East. When it is day in Mwimbe it is night in another country. The weight of the earth causes the sun to swing about and to pass over and go underneath, and the clouds are the roof.

Moon.—The moon went to bathe with the sun, but

when the moon got into the water the sun stole the moon's clothes and said: "Henceforth you will go naked, and you will only be able to show yourself for fifteen days in each month." This was because the sun was jealous of any rival in the sky.

(The sex of the moon is not specified.)

Stars.—The stars are the children of the sun and moon. There seems to be some knowledge of the difference between the planets and the stars, though there is no idea as to the origin of an eclipse.

Rainbow.—The rainbow rises from a dead man's head. It comes from the West, and it acts as a barrier to the rain, which always comes from the East.

Astronomy.—On the whole, the natives of Embu cannot be said to have much power of observation of stars and such matters—again, no doubt, owing to their utilitarian outlook. Nevertheless, there is some ground for saying that they know the difference between stars and planets, though they have little idea of the actual movements; nor are they interested in the constellations. Eclipses are remembered, and these, like comets, are regarded as being heralds of misfortune. The comet of 1910 caused considerable anxiety and alarm, until the death of King Edward was announced, whereupon all the natives accepted this as an adequate explanation of such a remarkable phenomenon. Otherwise no special attention is paid to the heavenly bodies, and nothing like astrology exists.

In connection with folk-lore, there are certain ideas

Tradition & Folk-Lore

about various animals and birds which lead to special treatment of them. For instance, the hornbill is said to have alarmed the people of Mwimbe on one occasion when they were in danger of a sudden attack, and on this account the hornbill is not eaten by any of that section. (Incidentally, this is no great deprivation, as anyone who has ever tried to make a meal off a hornbill will agree.)

The elephant is also regarded with considerable reverence and suspicion by the forest people. He is supposed to be related to human beings " because he has toes like a man, and because the cow-elephant suckles her calf like a woman." It is also sometimes said that no elephant will injure a pregnant woman. On account of this, a dead elephant counts as a corpse, and anyone touching it becomes unclean. This, however, does not prevent active elephant hunting, nor is ivory at all repellent to the native. The following is the ritual to be observed when a dead elephant or a piece of ivory is found by chance.

If a party is wandering about in the forest and they find a dead elephant, the first of the party says, " *Njogu yakwa !* " (my elephant), to stake his claim on the tusks. The second then says, " *Tumbura !* " (shares). The third says " *Ritho !* " (eyes). The fourth says, " *Maguru yakwa !* " (my feet). The fifth says, " *Thiriti yakwa !* " (my company or party)—and no one else has any claim at all.

Of these, Nos. 1 and 2 get a tusk each. Nos. 3, 4 and 5 get a goat when the ivory is sold.

Tradition & Folk-Lore

The tusks are taken to the village, but left outside while a *mundu mugo* is fetched. Nos. 1 and 2 provide a goat for the *mundo mugo* to kill. He kills it by suffocation, afterwards stabbing it in the throat with a knife. It is then skinned, and the skin remains the property of the *mundo mugo*. The contents of the stomach are mixed with black *dawa* (probably charcoal), and with the mixture all present rub their faces and hands. The flesh is eaten by the whole party. The intestines are emptied at the gate of the village, so that the party carrying the tusks are obliged to step in the stuff.

In the village the tusks are kept in a hut by themselves; no one goes there or sleeps there.

Every time the tusks are moved the ceremony has to be repeated. Before purification in this manner none of the party can eat with other people, being unclean.

CHAPTER XX

IN common with most African tribes the Embu natives have a very large number of questions and answers, which may be termed riddles. While varying in form, practically the same riddle can be found among all sections. They are generally known and by no means restricted to any one class. They are regarded as an amusing game and no special significance appears to attach to them. A man or woman will sometimes attain quite a reputation for them, and a halt on a journey or other leisure moment will form an occasion for an exhibition of ingenuity in this line.

The following may be regarded as a good sample list, though it is very far from being exhaustive.

The game is started by the questioner asking the equivalent of: " Are you ready? "—to which his respondent replies: " I am ready." These are termed *Ndaye*, or *Rogano*, the meaning of which seems to have no special significance.

Riddles

Questions	*Answers*
Ngwata Rogano (or Ndaye)	*Nagwata*
(Take a riddle)	(I take it)
The young men go, the old stay?	The river goes, the stones remain.
I had two goatskins, one dark and one light: I stretched them out to dry, and lo! they became one?	The earth and the sky.
You carry corpses to Emberre?	Sugar-cane. (There is none in Emberre, and the traveller there chews cane and spits out the pieces by the way.)
I walk round the hill, but my stick is curved, not straight?	A dog, with his tail.
I will go one way, and you will go another, and we will tie up our mother's clothes?	A door with its two posts.
My tree is so tall that you can never pluck the fruit at the top of it?	The highroad.
Why does your father hold your mother by the chin?	The roof pole of a hut which supports the beams.

Riddles

Questions	Answers
Your mother is big, and my mother is very small, but yet yours cannot grind corn like mine?	A wood-borer (which digs out fine powder).
I left something in a lake?	The spear of a warrior left upright in the bare ground.
Kibarabaru drives his cows from the top of the hill?	A razor, as it shaves the head.
(This name has no apparent meaning.)	
In the whole country there is nothing but whiteness?	A white robe.
What hangs down?	The " bell " bird.
Can you climb the *mganga*?	No, for it is the blade of a knife.
(Name peculiar and unexplained.[1])	
I come out at one door and go in at another?	A man goes to see his betrothed.
What is it that is bitter to the young men?	Not unripe bananas, but the *ndunguru* (a bitter ground berry).
I threw something and it went farther than an arrow?	A glance of the eye.

Riddles

Questions	*Answers*
Look at all these people standing round?	They are but the poles of the hut.
A cavern?	The mortar for extracting oil.
To milk my father's cow you will want a very big stool?	A bee-hive (hung in a tree so that it must be climbed to).
What is very finely attired?	A close-woven mat.
Here they say " *Huu !* " and there they say " *Huu !* " (thump)?	Two rams butting at each other.
There is a person who falls but never dies?	The moon.
My cattle feed everywhere?	The flies.
It has no relief?	A road which is never free of people.
My father's field is big, but there is only one head of millet in it?	The sky with the moon in it.
A centipede?	The Elders' Council with their staves.
There is a very big fire, but what shall we put on it?	The Sun.
I left it outside, and it turned to water?	A pot of fat.

Riddles

Questions	*Answers*
My father's field is large, but it has only one millet stalk on it ?	An old man's back with the backbone.
What feeds in my father's field after the harvest?	The sand-spider.
You follow something, but you cannot catch it?	The end of the road.

NOTE.—In connection with the above, it is very remarkable that many of the questions and answers given in the list are also to be found in the island of Mauritius. The creoles there have a similar game, which they term *sirandanes*, and this is widely popular there. Originating, no doubt, with the first negro slaves carried thither from East Africa, the questions and answers have survived translation not only from their original race, but even from their original language, so that it is possible now to find in Mauritius two people of pure Indian descent speaking creole French and asking the same riddles that are to be found among the primitive African tribes. The preliminary question in this case is " *Sirandane?* " to which the answer is " *Sampéque*," of which I have never been able to obtain any explanation. Some of the riddles are obviously taken from civilized life, but others are certainly derived from the original African form, of which the following are examples :—

Riddles

Questions	*Answers*
Mo banane, mo manze, zamais mo napas capa fini li ?	*Li grand cimin.*
(I keep on eating my banana, but I can never finish it?)	(The highroad.)
Dileau dibout ?	*Ene Lacanne.*
(Water upright ?)	(Sugar-cane.)
Dileau pendant ?	*Coco.*
(Water hanging ?)	(A coconut.)

NOTE

[1] But possibly meant to allude to the difficulty of overcoming the *mganga* (witch-doctor).

CHAPTER XXI

AN AUTOBIOGRAPHY

T HE following details are given, since they may be of interest, as the actual account of his life, given by an old man of remarkable personality. They represent the impressions made by the advent of civilization on the mind of an intelligent native. I have endeavoured throughout to keep as close as possible to the actual words used by the speaker, without including the inevitable questions and repetitions which would merely serve to obscure the course of the narrative. I have added nothing, and in talking to the speaker I carefully avoided any suggestion or leading question which might have influenced the trend of his story.

Chief Murunga, or *Kikono* (the Little Arm), was an important chief in Lower Mwimbe. He died just after the end of the war, at an advanced age for a native, probably over sixty. He retained his faculties and energies to an astonishing degree, and did not present the usual spectacle of hopeless senility which is the case with so many elderly natives. In middle life he lost his right arm at the elbow, which rather put a restraint on the activities which had previously brought him into prominence as an enterprising warrior and leader. He retained a considerable amount of influence, however, and was the chief of some five thousand people. He was a spirited old man, and had no sort of hesitation in speaking his mind to any audience; at times he was not above a little picturesque romance, as may be gathered from his entertaining, if decidedly doubtful, story of the raid on the Emberre cattle. Shrewd and tactful, he was quick to realize the power of the European, and to try to adapt himself to modern conditions; this, however, did not prevent periodical reversions to autocratic methods which were apt to take highly objectionable forms, such as tying up and half starving some personal enemy. Such " mistakes," as he gracefully terms them, tended to make him rather a handful for an administrative officer, though he was a fine and likeable old man.

" My father's name was Mtuanguo, my grandfather's was Gekunyu, and my great-grandfather's was Mbujo. Beyond that, I do not know the names of my family. My father, Mtuanguo, was not a big chief; he was a quiet man, who did not put himself forward, and so, though he was generally respected, he did not take a prominent place in society. His father, Gekunyu, however, was a very important man, especially in his old age, when he was one of the chief men in the local councils. He was a fine orator and also a brave warrior. His father, Mbujo, was a Mtheraka, and came to Mwimbe in his youth, I don't know why. He settled at the lower end of the hill, Kierra, some way from where my family has lived since.

An Autobiography

" My mother was a Meru woman. She came to be married to my father in the following way. There was a severe famine in Meru, and she and her brother came in a destitute state to my grandfather, Gekunyu, and were assisted by him. After many months the famine ceased, and the brother, my uncle, went home. But in the meantime my mother had fallen in love with my father, who was then a young warrior; my uncle objected, since it was not as good a match as he desired, but, since my family had been so kind to them, he gave his consent, and my father gave as dowry only three loads of chalk. My mother was a nice woman, better than the Mwimbe women.

" When I was born there was much more forest than there is now; there used to be large clumps of trees where there are now only one or two, if any at all. There was more game also, especially leopards, which were very bad; there were also many elephants, but the Akamba used to hunt them very much, as did our people too, though not so much; consequently they no longer come across the Tana as they did.

" My father told me that in his grandfather Mbujo's time there were plenty of cattle in our country. They had very long horns, and were quite different to any that we have now. But the Agumba came and carried off every one, so that we had no cattle at all. Also some cattle died from what we called *ruja*, a very fatal disease of the lungs. So the elders came together and decided on a special measure to prevent such a thing happening again. They took a fat sheep and burned it, and

229

cursed anyone who should pasture any cattle near our villages. So now we send our cattle to a distant part. [Note.—It is very likely that the precaution was taken against disease rather than raiders, since the Lower Mwimbe country is to this day most unhealthy for all stock.]

"When I was a child there was constant war going on between the Meru and our people; we were not troubled by the Masai or the Akikuyu, though they raided our neighbours in Upper Mwimbe on more than one occasion. At that time our principal chiefs were Mtuamtuanguo, and another man whose name was Ikura. The latter was a fine fighting man, and was also very cunning; he was a very fine chief. The greatest thing that he did was when he gained us some cattle, after we were left in poverty by the loss of the long-horned kind.

"He knew that there were many cattle in Emberre, so he assembled the young men, and said to them: ' Why should we remain poor, when we can get the cattle that we want by a little hard fighting in Emberre?' To this all the young warriors agreed, and a large party set out, under the leadership of Ikura, to raid the Emberre. Unfortunately the Emberre were ready for them, and they were all captured and tied up. But after four months Ikura escaped and returned home. He called all the elders together, and said that he had a plan for the recovery of the prisoners; they did not trust him very much after his failure, but his influence was great, and besides, what was there to do?

An Autobiography

So they listened to his plan. He made them bring him all the skins of cows that were to be found in the country, and he collected all the warriors that were left, with such elders as were still capable of fighting. He also took the only cow that was left in the country, and one fat sheep. Then he left home, and went to the boundary, the Thuchi, where the road crossed into Emberre. He sent to the Emberre, and told them that he had come to ransom all the prisoners, and that he had brought an enormous quantity of cattle for the purpose. He sent the fat sheep as a present, to show how well the Mwimbe stock was fed. The Emberre sent back to tell him to bring in the cattle. So he arranged to meet them at the border. They assembled on the hill-side, and he came up from the other direction. He made all his people walk on hands and knees, wearing the skins of the cows, so that in the distance they looked like cattle. In front, he drove the one cow, beating it all the way, so that it made a great noise. A messenger, who had been sent on before, called the attention of the Emberre to the herds which were approaching, saying : ' Don't you hear the cattle lowing?' As soon as they got anywhere near the border, Ikura sent and said that he was afraid of his cattle getting hurt by the thick bush that grew all along the road; the Emberre must cut a wider road before he could bring over such a great herd. So the Emberre made a fine road, right into the middle of their country.

"Then, on an appointed day, all the prisoners were

brought to the boundary, each man held by the man who had taken him. Ikura said that he was quite ready to pay generously, but that all the spears and swords must be given back with the prisoners. So all the weapons captured were brought and laid out, each one by its former owner. Then Ikura went over the border and began to bargain. As he expected, each man grew keen on his share of the ransom, and they neglected the prisoners; at last Ikura blew his war-horn, to summon the cattle, as he said. But the people inside the skins came as close as they could, and then charged down on the Emberre, who were taken by surprise. The prisoners took up their weapons, and the Emberre were slaughtered wholesale. All their cattle were carried off, which was very easy, since they had made a fine road at Ikura's suggestion. All our people returned home safe, and we had a great feast. Then Ikura built a very fine village, and he regulated our customs for us; after that he died. We still sing about him in our songs, for he was a very great chief. I don't remember him; I was only just born when he died.

"In those days there were always plenty of Swahili traders in our country. They came to buy ivory; they did not get slaves from us, but relied mostly on the Meru and the Akamba, I think, for those. But a half-brother of mine, who was on a visit to Meru, was sold as a slave, and has never come back. That was when I was a boy, so I don't suppose he will come back now.

"In my family there were four of us—my elder brother, myself, and then two sisters; but both my sisters are dead now. When I was old enough, I went through just the same ceremonies as the boys do now; but my sisters were let off lighter than the girls are nowadays. When I was a warrior, I fought against the Meru a lot, but never against the Chuka or people on the West. The weapons that I used were the old spear with the little blade, a sword like the present sword, and a shield much the same as the one used now. This was my own fancy; my father never used a shield; he always carried a bow and arrows, with sometimes a spear. But I never cared for the bow much, and of course after I had lost my arm I could not use one at all.

" This is the way that I lost my arm. We were having trouble among ourselves, and I was fighting with our neighbours, when someone shot me in the right wrist with an arrow which was covered with old stale poison. I pulled it out, but the head remained in, and as there was a lot of fighting going on I had to use my arm as best I could. The iron gradually worked up to the elbow, and my arm swelled up terribly. At last it got quite rotten, and fell off at the joint, with the bone; I was very glad, as it had given me a lot of trouble. At that time I was a middle-aged man, and led all the local warriors to battle; but I was not such a big chief as I am now.

" We fought chiefly with the Meru, who were driving us back from our old boundary, the Iraru; they were too strong for us, and we had to retreat, but only after a lot of fighting.

An Autobiography

"I got married just before I lost my arm; I have never had more than one wife at a time, and I was very fond of that one. I have recently married again, a young woman; she is a good creature, and takes care of me, but she is not as good as the first one: I suppose she would prefer a younger man, if I were not a chief.

"I first heard of the existence of white men when I was a warrior. They were then in the Akamba country, and I was told that the Masai were afraid of them. After that we heard that there was a great road along which the white men travelled. [NOTE.—Presumably the old caravan route to Uganda.] Then after some time we heard that they had arrived among the Akikuyu. But some while before that I had seen white men for the first time. Two of them came to our country from Tigania, where they had fought the Tigania because a servant of theirs had been killed. They had taken a lot of cattle, and their names were Mtuangondu and Mtuamburre. The first was a very tall man, much taller than you [that is, well over six feet], and the other was quite a small man. They came to our village and camped there for five days; one of their people was killed by some wandering Chuka, so they fought the Chuka, and took some of their cattle. Then they went to Meru, and later on they came back and camped near our village once more. They had a heap of ivory as big as a hill. After that they went to the Akamba country, but before they went they gave me two cows and ten goats.

234

An Autobiography

"It was not for a long time after that that I saw another white man. Then it was Kangange, at Embu. [Mr Horne, District Commissioner, probably about 1907.] We had heard that there was a white man in the Kikuyu country, and I went to see him out of curiosity. He promised that I should remain a chief, and he gave me a blanket with a picture of a lion on it, since I had told him that I was the Chief of all Mwimbe and Igoji as well. But there was trouble about my visit when I got home, and my people drove me away, because they did not wish to have anything to do with the white man. Later on, when Meru station was started, I went home again. Then you went to Tharaka, and on the way back my people attacked your party, because they did not want you to go through their country; I knew it was foolish, but they did not know much about white men then. No one was killed, but your people shot one man through the shoulder, and he was very ill for a long while. After that the Hawk Shooter [Mr Pigott, Acting District Commissioner, Embu, 1909] came and camped at my village; he was the first Government official to do so. Since then we have seen several other officials, and we know now that there are many white men; at first we thought that there were only a very few.

"Things have changed a lot lately. I prefer the present state of affairs, on the whole, but I can no longer go and take cattle from our neighbours, as we used to do, and that is a bad business for me, since I have only one arm, and am an old man, and can't work. If the Government went away again now, I should just have to follow, since I could no longer fight, and there are many of my old enemies still alive.

" My young men are better off than we were; but they are taking to drink, which is bad. We are richer and more comfortable than we used to be, owing to what people bring back when they return from work. But a terrible lot of new diseases have come about, and there are not as many young men as there used to be; soon we shall all be dead. But I am glad that the Government is here, and very likely the diseases will be forbidden to spread.

[Chief Kikono is given a present.]

" Thank you for the meat. I like telling you about old times since you are interested; I hope that next time I make a mistake you won't be as angry as you usually are. Now I will go home to my village."

NOTE.—Chief Kikono was speaking shortly after a serious epidemic of smallpox had been followed by a terrible outbreak of meningitis, hence, probably, his remarks about diseases.

CHAPTER XXII

THE natural history of the part of Kenya with which we have been dealing presents many features of great interest; for the influences which are responsible for the varied characteristics of the tribes in that region have also worked to produce a similar multiplicity of forms in the animals and plants. The great variation in altitude—from tropical plain to snow-line—in itself provides a kind of testing-ground, where each species has opportunity to try to adapt itself to heat or cold, and thereby spread farther. The fan-shaped system of rocky ravines which divides the country seems also to isolate the various ridges from each other, and no doubt to check the spread of particular forms. In consequence of these influences it is possible to find an almost incredible variety of entomological and botanical specimens, and the incidence of occurrence is most surprising. Fauna and flora being so largely interdependent, a collection in such a locality should naturally be as general as possible if it is to be of real value; the naturalist thus finds himself involved in so many branches that he would have to be a veritable Darwin to be able to cope with

237

them all. The geologist alone has little to contribute, for the country is almost entirely volcanic, so that this presents little opportunity for research, except for the specialized study of igneous action. But for the ornithologist, the entomologist and the botanist there is a fascinating field for inquiry; many years of work would be needed to exhaust the material presented. It will therefore be readily understood that, in the midst of official duties, and without adequate scientific resources such as a good microscope, I was able to do little more than collect a series of samples, in the hope that they would tempt some well-equipped scientist to embark upon a full survey of the region.

The larger animals are interesting, though not for the most part peculiar to Kenya. The elephant is the principal and occurs in considerable herds, which are mainly restricted to the forest; formerly far more common, they have been driven back into the less-frequented regions both by native trappers and by white hunters. Small parties still occasionally cross the Tana from the Mumoni country, but as a rule they are to be found only on the mountain slopes. Molestation has made them fierce and suspicious, and they attack on little or no provocation. One sees frequent instances of their well-known sagacity; indeed, were not the elephant well able to recognize his enemies and with-draw from dangerous spots, it is highly probable that he would have before now been extinct on Kenya. The old bulls in particular are extremely cautious and often display considerable intelligence when their suspicions are aroused. I knew of a case in which a solitary bull came along a road at night and approached within some fifty yards of a camp, presumably without being aware of its proximity, owing to the wind being in the wrong direction; he then discovered it and paused, swinging his weight from foot to foot, and then decided to retreat, which he did, walking backwards for some fifty yards before turning and making off through the bush, the whole episode being clearly recorded in his tracks in the dust. One can hardly resist the conclusion that past experience had in his mind connected human dwellings with guns and traps, and he therefore preferred to retreat along the path which he had already followed and therefore knew to be safe, while he kept his head toward the direction of possible danger.

The remaining herds on Kenya are now carefully protected, and they do little damage as a rule, except occasionally to a plantation near the forest; there seems no reason why they should not survive, therefore.

The elephant's relation, the rhinoceros, is much more troublesome, because far more stupid. Quite unable to take a hint that his presence is unwelcome, he insists on keeping to his original haunts, even when they are becoming populous and cultivated. Although really afraid of very little, he is suspicious and excitable, and an unaccustomed scent will often start him on a blundering, short-sighted charge without any other provocation; sooner or later, of course, this leads to his being shot. While one must sympathize with these quaint old survivals, it is nevertheless most annoying to have one's camp charged through in the middle of the night, or one's porters scattered on the line of march, with consequent damage to loads hurriedly thrown down. While unoccupied tracts of waste land will provide a refuge for some time to come, there can be little doubt that the poor old "rhino" is incompatible with civilization.

Buffaloes, on the contrary, have a much better idea of avoiding danger; like the elephants, they are largely withdrawing into the forests, and even in the last dozen years they have noticeably become more cautious, and less inclined to leave thick bush except by night. They breed of course much more rapidly than the pachyderms, and this has enabled the herds to recover very largely from the epidemics which have decimated them periodically in the past. Fierce and cunning, the buffalo is a dangerous quarry in thick bush, particularly when wounded; a surprisingly large proportion of accidents to big-game hunters come from following up a buffalo supposed to be dying.

Hippopotami and crocodiles are numerous in the larger rivers, and their numbers seem unlikely to decrease, though the latter could well be spared. It is a very common experience to find some bracelet, string of beads or other relic in the stomach of a dead crocodile, if the beast is of any size; the shooting of these dangerous and repulsive brutes is a ready road to popularity with the native, whose women-folk, in particular, are in constant danger, if they have to draw water from a river or large pool.

Lions and leopards are fairly common, but usually restrict their food to game; there are quite enough wild animals to keep them well fed, without attacking man, although the cattle are liable to suffer. An aged beast which can no longer follow game will sometimes turn man-eater, and lie in wait for children or women; the natives, however, are fairly plucky in their attitude towards these beasts, and will attack them with spears on occasion; the softer skin enables a heavy spear to penetrate it, so that the proposition is more hopeful than is the attack of an animal such as a rhino or buffalo. I knew of one occasion when an old woman gathering firewood suddenly saw a leopard in the grass, preparing to spring on her; summoning up all her strength, she struck it on the head with the narrow-bladed native axe which she was carrying, piercing the brain and killing the animal at once. She proudly brought the skull in to me with the axe, and I had great pleasure in rewarding the plucky old lady.

Cats of several varieties are troublesome, in stealing chickens and so forth; they show astonishing vitality, and unless mortally wounded, or very effectually trapped, they almost always contrive to get away with their booty.

An interesting creature is the aard-vark, or anteater, which, though numerous, is hardly ever seen; the large holes which they dig are very common (and annoying) features of the roads throughout the district. In shape something like a large rabbit, but with bat-like ears, long snout and strong talons, they are entirely nocturnal; while their acute hearing sends them underground at the slightest sound. Consequently they are very rarely captured, especially as their remarkable digging power enables them to keep ahead of even a vigorously wielded shovel and pick.

Wart-hog, wild pig and baboons are responsible for considerable damage to plantations, the last being particularly mischievous. Travelling in large parties of several dozen, under the leadership of an old chief, they will settle into a patch of maize and pull off almost every cob, throwing about and wasting far more than they eat. Although rumoured to be occasionally dangerous (as they well might be, with their great strength and formidable jaws), I never knew of an instance of them molesting human beings. On one occasion I came on a raiding party in the tree-tops in the forest near my station, and I shot the leader, to drive them away. He fell with a crash, uncomfortably like an old man, and the rest of the troop became most excited and indignant; they followed me along in the branches almost overhead, and looked so threatening that I quite thought they meant to drop down and attack me; and as I had only a rook-rifle I was decidedly uneasy. By shooting four more I kept them

Natural History

at a little distance, although they followed me to the edge of the forest; probably they would not have ventured to attack me, but at the time I felt far from sure of this. They are very intelligent and audacious, and know well who is likely to be dangerous. An assistant of mine came upon an isolated native hut outside which two children wept disconsolately, while a large baboon placidly helped himself to the family dinner in the pot in front of him. They also certainly recognize, and fear, a gun of any kind.

Hyenas are very numerous, and fill a definite position in society as the universal undertakers; in spite of their very powerful jaws they are cowardly beasts, and I never knew them to attack a human being on Kenya, though I have found instances of this elsewhere. They will, however, sometimes try to drag away a native sleeping near a fire, but no doubt in such cases they believe him to be a corpse. Like the baboons, they are impudent marauders; a small one was once killed in my camp after having got his head firmly wedged in the enamelled jug into which the cows were milked—an extraordinary object as he blundered about the camp in the firelight with the jug jammed over his ears.

The forest holds many interesting animals in addition to those already mentioned; as one grows accustomed to, and familiar with, these great tree-covered stretches of country one begins to realize how much goes on in them which is entirely unsuspected at first. Among the forest-dwellers proper should perhaps be mentioned, first, the giant forest hog. This monster of his tribe seldom leaves the shelter of the great trees, and many people who have lived long near his habitat have nevertheless failed to catch a glimpse of him. Occasionally, however, he emerges and tries a little plundering in a potato-field or native garden which is near enough to the edge of the forest for him to dare the risk. I was lucky enough to fall in with one such occasion, and was able to secure the marauder, which proved to be a record, standing 3 feet 10 inches at the withers, and measuring 7 feet 4 inches from snout to tail.

Of similar retiring habit, and less objectionable taste, the bongo should be mentioned next. This remarkably fine animal is by no means rare in the forest, but is so very shy and wary that it is quite exceptional to find anyone who has even seen one. The very early morning is the best time to look for it, but great patience and study of the animal's habits are essential to success. I was most unfortunately forestalled in the pursuit of a fine specimen by a lion, which killed and partly ate the bongo while I was camped impotently a couple of miles away. I secured the head—a record—but naturally took little interest in the second-hand trophy. In a somewhat similar way I found by chance a fairly fresh buffalo head, lying where the owner had died, in the forest; measurement showed it to be almost a record, but I was glad to accept a good offer for it.

Several other interesting animals are occasionally to be found in the forest; the rare Isaacs Duiker, with a curious goat-like profile, is to be met with if one is lucky; I shot a nice specimen by accident, not knowing what I had secured until I examined the animal, since I had fired under the impression that it was a common species, and had been actuated by hunger rather than science. But it has always been my experience that one's best trophies are secured practically by accident; some fluke secures an animal of exceptional interest, when perhaps a long and exhausting chase after a carefully selected quarry ends in disappointment.

Among the forest-dwellers must be mentioned the mysterious " Kitanga," which is so far unrecorded in any list of trophies. This beast seems to be well authenticated by native account, and would seem to be a forest cheetah; the people describe it as much like a lion, but with the habits of a leopard; it is said to have non-retractile claws, and to be exceptionally fierce. I have seen a skin of the beast, which was to me indistinguishable from that of the cheetah of the plains; the only point of interest in it was the very definite affirmation by the natives that the animal had been killed in the forest fifty miles or more from any spot where a cheetah had ever been heard of. There would certainly seem to be a beast of the nature of a forest-dwelling cheetah to be found on

245

Natural History

Kenya, though it sounds unlikely, in view of the profound modifications that the animal's habits would have to undergo to render him fit for life under such conditions.

The forest teems with interesting matter for the zoologist, and a really careful and prolonged study of the region would surely yield many new forms; in addition to mammals, there are many interesting fields for research, such as birds and lizards, while bats should also not be neglected. An endeavour might also be made to secure some living specimens of the more interesting and rare animals; there is no reason to suppose that it would prove difficult to rear and transport a half-grown specimen of, say, the bongo or the forest hog. I made some effort to secure such specimens, but was successful only in the case of the Colobus monkey, of which I captured a half-grown male. He proved an interesting and very intelligent pet, though he never grew very tame; still, he developed a surprising amount of sense in the way in which he would indicate the particular leaves which he wanted included in his food; so clear were his explanations, indeed, that I was greatly helped in getting him accustomed to a more varied diet, with a view to his journey to the Zoological Gardens; this was successfully accomplished, but unfortunately he died of lung trouble in the succeeding autumn. Poor beast, I wonder whether his real scientific value justified his exile from his native forest?

The animals of the forest have been little studied,

and there is a virgin field for research for a naturalist who will devote time and study to the subject; it may be as well to add that he should be sound in nerve, as continued life in the forest is perhaps of all solitary conditions of existence the most trying to the nerves.

CHAPTER XXIII

NATURAL HISTORY (*continued*)

THE insects of Kenya form a most absorbing and astonishing field for research, since very few parts of the world could rival the bewildering variety of forms which confront the collector. Not only do the variations of temperature and vegetation lead to a wonderful range of species; there is a special fascination in observing the same insect as it appears in its various forms, from the perfect example, living under conditions which suit it well, to the dwarfed or maldeveloped struggler which is trying to preserve existence under conditions quite unfavourable to it. South-East Kenya would be a happy hunting-ground for any naturalist who wished to observe the modifications brought about in any species by change of environment. It is, of course, impossible to dogmatize without the fullest evidence and an ample collection of specimens; but there seems to be some reason for saying that it is quite possible to find forms where the insect in one locality lives through its full cycle, while not far away, under less favourable conditions, it does so only in a stunted and immature form; and still farther away it possibly fails altogether to complete the life cycle. As a kind of natural laboratory

248

or testing-ground for evolutionary theories, this country must be ideal.

Without pretensions to scientific work, I made such collection as I was able, being greatly encouraged thereto by the constant sympathy and appreciation of the authorities of the South Kensington Museum; my only regret was that I could not afford the time necessary to follow up the very interesting lines of investigation which they in some cases suggested to me.

The majority of the insects of the slopes of Kenya are, of course, common species, and the principal factor of interest in their cases is distribution; but I also found numerous specimens which could not be identified, and which were very possibly immature, modified or primitive forms of some known insect.

Mosquitoes were numerous, but no new forms appeared among my specimens; nevertheless, I was frequently puzzled at the erratic appearance of certain types; in particular there would seem to be some local influence at work which tends towards segregation of the sexes[1]; in several cases I found males in profusion with scarcely a female, while elsewhere, or at other times, the position would be reversed. This was certainly far more noticeable than it is in any other locality of which I am aware.

The dreaded tsetse is fairly common in the lower country, and is no doubt largely responsible for shortage of cattle in Emberre; but sleeping sickness among humans is happily unknown in that part. As

Natural History

I have noticed in other countries in Africa, the distribution of Glossina is very largely dependent on the season; one year they will be found in quantities all along some river-bed, while in the following year they will be almost absent, even in the corresponding season; there seems to be little doubt that they depend very largely on rainfall and the consequent vegetable growth. This fact makes one slightly sceptical of the value of the usual " tsetse map " with clearly defined boundaries marked out in red; an exceptional year might well render such a map a dangerous trap for the unwary cattle-owner who trusted its definition too implicitly.

A most interesting feature of the forest insects is the blood-sucking Hæmatopota; at certain times of the year these voracious flies occur in innumerable swarms along the margin of the forest; so ferocious are they that, should one get among them on a horse or mule, one must wheel round and gallop out again to avoid the animal being driven crazy by their painful bites. This raises the interesting point of their natural food; such ravenous swarms must require large supplies of animal victims to meet their needs. Yet when one examines the position one can only say that the supply is extremely scanty; they must take their chance of an occasional elephant or buffalo, with possibly a rare chance at a bongo or forest hog; in which case they must range very widely to secure even a periodical meal. The birds and the long-haired Colobus monkey are too well protected to be attacked; while the very painful nature of the bite renders it quite impossible for the insect to feed undetected by its host.

If this is puzzling in the case of *Hæmatopota alluaudi*, still more is it when we come to consider *Hæmatopota distincta*, the smaller and less common species to be found on the higher slopes of the mountain. The latter begins at some 10,000 feet, and is to be found right up to 12,000 feet, and even higher. Seeing that at the latter altitude any warm-blooded animal is practically not to be found, it is a problem what the fly can find to feed upon. At 13,000 feet I found them still far from rare, and apparently very well pleased to secure a supply of blood; and yet, with the exception of one or two birds and a small rat-like creature, I could see no trace of any source of possible food supply. Again, it is astonishing that such a comparatively small insect should be able to stand a daily range of temperature from tropical sunshine by day to many degrees of frost by night.

Ants of numerous varieties are common, persistent and astonishingly efficient. The termite, or so-called white ant, is responsible for an immense amount of damage every year; I have tried numerous remedies and cannot say that I found any of them very efficacious. Various preparations exist which are said to render material ant-proof, and they do seem to repel the insect to some extent; personally, however, I am prepared to believe that, failing anything more attractive, such as saddlery, furniture or books, they would eat chilled steel.

Natural History

The ferocious red ants, the *siafu*, are also most active and disconcerting visitors. Travelling in a well-organized column, they are most determined and aggressive; any living creature in their way has to make a rapid escape or be driven mad by bites, as has happened even in the case of horses, when shut up in a stable and unable to escape. Making a well-defined track an inch or so in width, it is only with the greatest difficulty that they can be deterred from following it; hot ashes, or quantities of snuff, will turn them aside for a while, but they will find a way round and continue the same line of march eventually. Another astonishing detail is their fidelity to the same track for each move. Since they seem to migrate every six months from one nest to another some hundreds of yards away, it is very curious that they should follow back the same track as they used in their previous move; I certainly knew of two tracks which were faithfully followed for four successive migrations, although the whole surface of the ground had been completely altered in the interval; one track, indeed, led diagonally across my new kitchen, the existence of which merely led to a diversion along the two sides back to the old path again. These insects form an absorbingly interesting study, but unfortunately the trail often ends in thick bush, where their natural ferocity makes it very awkward to follow them up. Certainly they possess an astonishing amount of organization, while the unanimity with which they will swarm unobtrusively all over a victim, and then attack simultaneously, is almost incredible.

Natural History

Vegetation shows as much response to unusual climatic conditions as do insects; the whole area of South-East Kenya is one great testing-ground for the innumerable varieties of plants to be found there. While a most interesting collection of wild specimens might be made in the locality, perhaps an even more promising line for research lies in the effect of locality upon apparently well-established species of domestic plants. One can find a patch where English conditions are reproduced fairly closely in the matter of soil and temperature; with some shading through the hot hours of sunshine, there is little difference from an English summer. And yet look at the results which are obtained! Sow seed from some reputable firm in Europe, and continue to plant each season, using the seed from the previous crop; do this for, say, four generations and examine the result. For instance, lettuce of a well-established cos variety will produce, in the first season, a beautiful, crisp, close-hearted specimen, that would win a prize at any agricultural show. Let it run to seed, and plant these; you will get a lettuce, certainly, but a lanky, straggling sort of thing; collect its seeds and sow these, and you will have something that is scarcely recognizable as a lettuce; while with the next generation you arrive at a plant some three feet in height, looking much like a dandelion crossed with a thistle, and carrying small tough leaves at intervals up its stout stem; embryo thorns garnish its ribs, and a thick milky latex of noticeably soporific qualities can be freely obtained from its fractures.

Natural History

Other plants show equal response to local conditions, though each in its own way; thus the carnation grown from seed flourishes wonderfully, but gradually the wide range of colours diminishes, until the pink-flecked white variety outlives them all; the dahlia, on the contrary, will go on crossing until the variety of colours is bewildering. The snapdragon tends to produce only the Delilah variety, with throat of different colour to the hood; and the geranium aims steadily at vermilion. Even more interesting is the sweet-pea; the startling readiness with which it will in the second generation develop quite unexpected colours renders it certain that Bateson's experiments in allelomorphism in these plants would produce most interesting results. There is a marked tendency to revert to purple, and the bicolour type seems the stronger; which is much as might be expected, though de Vries' work makes it difficult to understand the vigour of the Delilah Antirrhinum, which is nevertheless seemingly well established.

Among vegetables the same unwelcome inclination to develop inconvenient ancestral tendencies is manifest. Celery and asparagus adopt as their model the bootlace; the radish, on the contrary, takes as its ideal the football; and as in each case a watery stringiness replaces the desirable natural flavour, the amateur gardener feels disheartened.

Almost endless other examples might be quoted of odd and unexpected behaviour of plants under local conditions, and the problem at once arises, What is the particular influence at work? One can largely eliminate soil and temperature, since these can be arranged to reproduce very much the European characteristics, when one has such a range of heights to select from. The outstanding difference would seem to be the rays of the sun; just as these have a very different effect upon the photographic plate on the Equator from that produced in England (even when the exposure meter registers the same figure), so the English plants are similarly affected, one can only conclude.[2] Certainly Kenya results cannot be reproduced in England under hothouse conditions, even with artificial manure or other stimulus to growth and unusual development. There would seem to be some steady influence at work which affects all the products of the temperate zone when transferred to the Equator; and to it must presumably be attributed the nervous exhaustion, insomnia, irritability and lack of control (and even suicide in extreme cases) which are to be observed in so many of the white residents who have been too long without change; just as the same influence affects the European dog in deterioration of sporting qualities, and the European fruit or vegetable in flavour and type. It would be of great interest to carry out a series of experiments in which various patches of seed were grown under shade, under coloured glass, under solutions designed to filter out certain rays, and finally in the open; careful comparison of the results through several generations should admit of very instructive deductions as to the influence of the particular light affecting the various patches. With these experiments might be combined tests on the lines of the patient work of Lord Avebury in testing the sensitivity of ants to light; the termites, the larvæ of mosquitoes, and numerous wood-boring insects should afford good material for experiment. I had planned some rudimentary tests on these lines, but unfortunately the Kaiser had arranged for my occupation otherwise.

The south-east slopes of Kenya offer a wonderfully wide field for research; my foregoing remarks are made in the hope that leisured and trained scientists will be tempted to follow the track diffidently suggested by a busy official.

The mapping of the glaciers of Kenya was one of my ambitions, but unfortunately I never had the opportunity or time to spare for this arduous task; my highest point was nearly 15,000 feet, but I was forced to return owing to lack of equipment and time, and such work as I was able to do in the way of survey-ing has since been quite eclipsed by that of Dr Arthur. The collections that I made on that occasion were sent to the South Kensington Museum, while I retain for my own satisfaction the memory of the truly wonderful view of distant Kilimanjaro from the upper slopes of Kenya, as it glimmered like a flamingo's feather in the light of the rising sun, after a miserable night which we spent huddled over a fire of heather roots, with the temperature many degrees below freezing, and our heat-accustomed lungs and skins trying in vain to adjust themselves to the startling change. I believe myself to have been the first white man to see this view; my nearer acquaintance with Kilimanjaro was made when I was in command of a battery in action in the plains beneath. The two great mountains are now under one flag, and there is something fitting in the thought that these two timeless giants are no longer vexed with the squabblings over an international boundary between them.

See the author's article, " The South-East Face of Mount Kenya," in *The Geographical Journal,* June 1918.

NOTES

[1] " The imago emerges from the pupa during the late afternoon, after which the females are ready for fertilization by the males. These latter can sometimes be seen in large numbers, while but few females are observed, which is supposed to be characteristic of the breeding period " (*Manual of Tropical Medicine*, Cestellani and Chalmers).

[2] " When bright sunshine falls upon a leaf, about a quarter of its radiant energy is absorbed. A much larger relative amount is taken up when the light is less bright; in a strong diffuse light, such as that from a clear northern sky, the absorption amounts to about 96 per cent. of the incident energy" (*Vegetable Physiology*, Reynolds Green).

CHAPTER XXIV

PRESENT & FUTURE

AFTER the foregoing survey of the primitive institutions of this group of tribes it may perhaps be useful to add some observations and speculations as to the probable line of development of these people under modern conditions.

An outstanding feature of the case is one which is common to most African tribes, but which has nevertheless perhaps received less attention than its importance merits — I allude to the extent to which African psychology must be regarded from the point of view of crowd psychology. Modern conditions in civilized communities have produced a society where individuals are in constant close contact, but it is very doubtful if this is so much the case as it is in an African village. The native lives almost perpetually in a crowd; not only is his own family always about him, but almost any action is done in company with others. He grows up in the midst of the children of the village, he undergoes his initiation into manhood in company with a number of his fellows, he goes out to look for work in a crowd, and with that crowd he is paid off or deserts; in old age he reaches the Elders' Council, and once more forms a unit of a party. If this is the case with the man, still more is it so with the woman; he may occasionally make a journey, when he may possibly be alone for an hour or two; she, however, is probably hardly ever alone for more than half-an-hour throughout her life. It may perhaps be said that something of the sort is also the case with industrial workers in large cities; but these have at any rate the possibility of withdrawing themselves in contemplation of the printed page; the native has no such resource, and leads an entirely exterior life.

This condition must obviously have a profound effect on his mentality and his attitude towards life; and in dealing with him it is most important to remember that one is constantly confronted with the psychology of the crowd, rather than that of the individual; a very slight acquaintance with the principles of sociology will suffice to emphasize the importance of this distinction.

The student of Gustav le Bon will find much in Africa to which his principles and analysis apply with startling force, though perhaps on an elementary scale. It is a misfortune that most Europeans who come into contact with primitive Africans are of necessity men who have led solitary, self-reliant, individualistic lives, and who are therefore specially handicapped in an endeavour to realize a mentality in which the individual becomes largely submerged in the crowd, and on which public opinion exercises an almost overwhelming force.

It is this outlook which is responsible for the greater

part of the actions of natives; it upholds native law and custom, or, again, it may serve to hasten their downfall when "fashion" sets against them; it influences a gang of labourers to go and seek some particular employment, and a slight veering of the wind may also lead the same gang to desert precipitately for no real reason. Always the individual finds it extremely difficult to act in defiance of the opinion of the crowd.

This carries with it the corollary that the individual when separated from the crowd becomes conspicuously weak and wavering; accustomed to follow the herd, he is bewildered when he has to act and decide for himself, and make a choice between his own old custom and the alien ways of strangers around him. This accounts for the deplorable readiness of the travelled native to abandon his own salutary beliefs in favour of the vague lawlessness of town communities; and it also explains why a group of entirely satisfactory native Christians will prove so very unsatisfactory when scattered as isolated individuals.

Considering now the position of these primitive tribes in face of the sudden coming of European civilization, it must be remembered that this represents to them absolute and complete revolution; in almost every phase of life we are radically altering the native's established methods and beliefs. In administration we give him entirely new and foreign criminal and civil laws; in social life we substitute money for barter, and introduce him to clothing, education, the wage system, and a whole host of other startling innovations; while in the unseen world we amaze him with the offer of a creed which gives him a glimpse of an unknown world and a future life, while it strikes at the root of all his old beliefs. And this breathless rush through stages of progress which have taken many centuries for other races is being made willy-nilly under the forced guidance of the European, whether the native wishes it or not. No doubt it will be contended that this is inevitable, and that the white man is entitled to force his views on the native since he knows best what is good for the subject race. The same argument has been used to support the Bolshevist movement, and yet other nations resisted it on the grounds that they preferred to choose for themselves. Can the African be altogether blamed when he shows some signs that he regards himself as being unduly hustled?

Be this as it may, we are undeniably introducing profound changes, and tearing up deep-rooted ideas, at a most precipitate rate; and with such far-reaching changes must come a new orientation for the native outlook. As Gustav le Bon says: " When a faith ends, a revolution begins "[1]; it is a dangerous thing to destroy one belief without substituting another for it.

The tribes with which we have been dealing are in many ways decidedly intelligent and promising material; but a serious error is often made in believing superficial acquirements to be deep changes. The native may, and frequently does, adopt European ways to a very large extent, and he may seem to have acquired also the European outlook; but it is highly probable that under stress this will vanish like breath from a mirror, leaving the old basic prejudices as motives of conduct. I knew of a case in South Africa where an elderly missionary couple brought up a native baby almost as their own son, only to see him one day, when he was about eighteen, declare his independence and his determination to return to his own people; which he did, becoming a specially unattractive and savage-looking inhabitant of the native location. This is perhaps an extreme instance, but somewhat similar cases will occur to anyone of African experience.

Such examples are eloquent of the danger of mistaking a surface veneer for a complete change. If a permanent foundation is to be secured upon which a new native social organization can rest, it must surely be evolved on lines which admit of adaptation of old laws and traditions, rather than by the forcible application of completely alien ideas. The Germans in East Africa tried, with the usual Prussian spirit, to turn the African into a reproduction of a European agricultural serf; he was to be allowed to develop, but only along approved lines; much would be done for him, but solely on condition that he learnt the lessons taught him. Native authority, individuality and tradition were all rooted out as far as possible, and a carefully thought-out, soulless Prussian bureaucracy was aimed at, which would have been equally applicable, or inapplicable, to Chinese or Americans.

The result was that a rapid and serious degeneration

262

set in; the old standards were broken down, and the new ones did not replace them, since they entirely lacked the respect and support of the people themselves; the population was being speedily reduced to a mass of sheep-like serfs who lacked all power of independent judgment. They were told to do, or to refrain from doing, a number of things; and failure to obey led to prompt punishment; outside the rules, however, no guidance of native tradition or European law or ethics controlled them, and they merely drifted along the path of wanton inclination, with the result that they were rapidly degenerating, both physically and morally.

Such a result is obviously disastrous. A race cannot advance upon lines which eliminate individual character and self-respect; it is essential for the native to have a standard to which he adheres from his own belief and freewill instead of a set of forcibly maintained rules which fail to cover more than the elements of social organization, and which he will rapidly reduce to the basic commandment: " Thou shalt not be found out."

This may be perhaps an obvious ideal; it is, however, depressingly difficult to see what measures should be employed in practice to advance towards it. The Elders' Councils are utilized as far as possible; the people are consulted on measures which affect them, and native authority is supported and developed wherever it proves trustworthy. Nevertheless, progress is deplorably slow; corruption and inefficiency are so common that there is a standing temptation to fall back upon hard-and-fast European methods of control in order to cope with the rapidly developing situation, where native society is speedily disintegrating under the force of advancing civilization.

Happily the African has a mentality which is not a complicated or highly strung one; he is severely practical and matter-of-fact even in his superstitions, for these are, after all, only misapplied experience when analysed. He threads his way through the maze of ceremonial uncleanness not from any obscure spiritual motive, but because he believes that prompt calamity would follow infringement. Abstract ideas such as patriotism or love of liberty appeal to him only in concrete form; he objects to losing his land or being shut up in jail, but the principles on which such transactions take place are quite beyond his grasp; so he is perfectly ready to help to filch his neighbour's land, or shut his brother up in jail, if it seems to be to his advantage.

It is this habit of mind that accounts largely for the native's attitude towards religion : Islam seems reasonable enough, except for its absurd refusal to allow intoxicants; Christianity is an attractive, easy-going creed, except for its deplorably narrow-minded view of polygamy. So he adopts one or the other, but with a saving clause which exempts him from the objectionable doctrines, and is disappointed and hurt when the professors of the creed regard him as an unsatisfactory convert: surely half-a-loaf is better than no bread?

Such a mentality is unlikely to prove fertile soil for

any great popular movement; Panislamism will have to offer something more tangible than the delights of Paradise before it can proclaim a Holy War in Kenya; and equally, an armed rising against European authority could only succeed for a brief space under some such doctrine as the invulnerability of all those treated by some medicine-man; the first few casualties would discredit the power of the charm, and any subsequent resistance would be owing to fear of punishment rather than continued faith in the movement.

What then might furnish grave administrative difficulties among these tribes? Here the conditions of crowd mentality seem to supply the answer. It is quite possible that combination might have serious developments; passive resistance and the boycott are both weapons which the native would very readily grasp and use. With a definite object in view, and plausible leaders to advocate it, the Kenya tribes might well prove capable of resistance which would bring administrative and industrial machinery to a complete standstill. Such a movement would be far harder to deal with than an armed rising which could be answered with machine-guns, and yet, with evil counsellors, the object of the one might be quite as reprehensible and inadmissible as that of the other.

The question of leadership is an important one. It must be remembered that these people largely lack natural leaders; the enormously wealthy chiefs to be found around Lake Victoria, or the respected dynasties of the coast Arabs, are without counterpart on the slopes of Kenya; and this would render it the easier for an upstart to gain a large following. An aristocracy of either wealth or birth makes at any rate for security against sudden and tempestuous popular movements; where such is practically non-existent, there is less for the ambitious demagogue to overcome in his seizure of popular power.

Sound education would seem to be the best safeguard; a channel of development for the enterprising, with some definite and attainable goal to be reached. Abstract theoretical instruction, resulting in the production of swarms of inefficient clerks for whom no work can be found, would be entirely pernicious; but sound education, on industrial lines, with a view to meeting the great existing demand for craftsmen, must surely have the approval of everyone. There is no apparent reason why the local native should not be educated up to take his place as mason, carpenter, mechanic, or a host of other avocations now carried on in most cases by doubtfully desirable Asiatics or extremely expensive Europeans.

One feature of German administration which is at any rate well worthy of imitation was the excellent education which they were beginning to give the native. Their frank insistence on a complete colour bar when dealing with Indians made the latter reluctant to go to German East Africa; it was therefore necessary to develop the African, and as a result the German schools were beginning to turn out really capable and well-trained artisans and mechanics. The constantly growing demand for such men led to their rapid absorption, and there was thus ample opening in a really useful field, for the enterprising and well-behaved native.

The introduction of European novelties in the form of tools and appliances presents some difficulties; it is by no means easy to tell whether a newly introduced appliance will be well received and rapidly adopted, or regarded with lethargic dislike. Clothing and blankets, for instance, were taken up with almost regrettable alacrity, while various tools, notably knives, were also eagerly welcomed. Other articles, however, are even now rare in the native homestead although easily acquired and far preferable to the native equivalent; cooking-pots, plates and lamps are fair examples. The explanation of this probably lies in the question of the sex concerned in the using; the African woman (like her sisters elsewhere) is usually far more conservative than the man. He will readily exchange his goat-hide cloak for a blanket, but she will cling to her skin petticoat in preference to cloth, even when she has the chance of the latter, unless of course she has become detribalized. He will buy a steel knife to replace his native-made iron one, but she will continue to cook in the old pottery vessels rather than the imported metal ones. She has got as far as a metal hoe for her weeding, and is open to conviction in the matter of new varieties of beads and such things, but she dislikes anything that entails a change of time-honoured custom.

Present & Future

For this reason a bicycle will be regarded as less of an innovation than a plough, although the latter would seem much more obvious and acceptable. But the bicycle is merely a new and exciting form of travelling which does not upset any established prejudices; the plough, on the contrary, means the readjustment of all the traditional ideas of cultivation; large fields instead of the old small patches (with consequent confusion as to the woman's duties and rights in the crop); draught animals to work, instead of the immemorial hoe and digging-stick; and an initial expense which entails collaboration to an extent which is quite alien to these primitive people. As a contrast may be mentioned the ready acceptance of ploughs by the more advanced tribes farther west, who have to some extent the elaborate social organization of the Baganda, and who therefore find much less difficulty in organizing communal enterprise under the leadership of a powerful chief.

Such aspects should not be overlooked when considering education and development of the native; it is useless to try to thrust upon him some unwelcome novelty, even though it may be a genuine improvement on his own methods; a much easier line of advance will be to encourage him to adopt such innovations as appeal to him, and use these as a means of education towards the establishment of less attractive novelties.

For a long time to come a paternal method of administration will probably be necessary; the Kenya native finds it very difficult to conceive of an abstract authority behind the individual with whom he is dealing. He has a vague idea of a Government which issues orders to administrative officers, but he nevertheless regards a particular official as personally responsible for any new method or system introduced. He is quite incapable of grasping such a situation as an energetic manager struggling to save a derelict plantation; he merely regards the manager as close-fisted and exacting. Still less can the African mind rise to the conception of a superior court which on principles of strict law and procedure upsets the decision of the district officer on some criminal case. The officer concerned told the prisoner that he had done wrong and would go to prison; now this vague authority in the background says that the man is to be set free; presumably, therefore, he had done no wrong. Everybody knows that he committed the offence, indeed he admitted it; what then can one make of these extraordinary Europeans who can't even agree whether such a simple act is right or wrong? It is a most exceptional native who can grasp the idea of such scrupulously fair procedure, that some mistake which prejudices the case for the accused may necessitate the quashing of an otherwise unexceptionable sentence.

The application of the law to the native, and the method of punishing the offender, present great problems; it seems very difficult to devise a system in which the reformative element shall outweigh the

Present & Future

deterrent aspect of punishment; almost any attempt on such lines leads to an improvement of jail conditions which may make prison positively popular. Where no social stigma is attached to penal servitude, a prison must be made unpleasant in some way; and already jail life is looked upon without much distaste, except in the case of a long sentence, when the native feels the continued confinement, loss of amusements and absence of female society very trying. There are the two purely deterrent forms of punishment, hanging and flogging. The first probably has little effect on the native mind in general, though public execution would certainly enormously increase the impression made by a death sentence. If execution on the scene of the crime be considered inadmissible, it is arguable if capital punishment achieves its purpose at all. Flogging undeniably has a marked effect, and since the native certainly does not consider himself degraded at all thereby, either as executant or recipient, it loses much of its objectionable nature.[2] At all events, until the science of criminology has made far more progress in Africa, the juvenile delinquent will receive much more benefit from a sound caning than from a prison, reformatory or compulsory industrial school, which only too often may be in reality merely a university of crime. The present proportion of juvenile recidivism is a reproach to our methods; there is an urgent need for another Lombroso who will deal with the peculiar aspects of crime and punishment in Africa.

Present & Future

The effect of the war upon the native was in almost every way most unfortunate, quite apart from the loss of life and damage to prosperity. It is true that he gained an enormously increased respect for the power and resources of the mysterious European, which must serve as a great deterrent to any idea of armed movements ; but against that advantage must be set the effect upon the native mind of seeing the previously all-wise European embark upon a bitter and prolonged war of an extent and duration utterly beyond African experience. Quite without comprehension of the principles involved, and unsupported by ideas of patriotism or glory, the native found himself involved in a chaos of death, starvation, disease and general misery, which he could only regard in much the same light as an earthquake or a cyclone, excepting always that the European was somehow responsible for it all.

To the more intelligent such a revelation must have had a marked effect in making them doubtful whether the white man's ways were really preferable to their own. Of necessity, in a campaign very many ugly things have to be done, while the stripping off of many of the restraints of civilized life left the ruling race only too often in a most unprepossessing light. It is to be hoped that the simple philosophy and ready forgetfulness of the African will speedily eradicate such recollections from his mind.

It must also be remembered that the " blessings of civilization " are not in practice by any means as obvious as some simple-minded folk would like to believe. It can be said with fair accuracy that among the tribes with which we have been dealing there is, in their uncontaminated society, no pauperism, no paid prostitution, very little serious drunkenness, and on the whole astonishingly little crime; while practically everyone has enough to eat, sufficient clothing, and an adequate dwelling, according to the primitive native standard. Of what civilized community can as much be said? Certain outstanding benefits we have undoubtedly conferred, notably the abolition of the ghastly slave trade; we have also by means of vaccination wiped out the disastrous epidemics of smallpox which devastated the country periodically, even up to the time that most of these notes were made. We have also done something to free the native mind from much benighted superstition, and to introduce sounder ideas of fair play and self-respect; many material benefits have also followed white rule which have done much for the comfort and health of the African. Nevertheless, from the point of view of abstract happiness, one can hardly blame the older people for turning their glances backwards. The colt galloping about a field must some day be broken to saddle or harness if he is to justify his existence, but it is idle to pretend that he is thereby made happier. Progress is inevitable, and no race can nowadays live inside a ring-fence; the problem is how to guide that progress so that it may be along sound lines, with the inevitable accompanying evils deprived as far as possible of their pernicious results. A grave responsibility for the future development of a race rests upon all those, whatever their calling may be, who are taking part in the great changes now influencing the tribes of Kenya.

NOTES

[1] " Les révolutions qui commencent sont en réalité des croyances qui finissent " (*Psychologie des Foules*).

[2] " Incarceration in jail may be said to involve no punishment for negroes, but rather gives to the idle and vicious desired rest, and, in the eyes of their racial friends, elevates them to the dignity of martyrs. We seriously advise, therefore, for many obvious reasons, the infliction of corporal punishment upon all freedmen who commit offences not subject to long terms of imprisonment " (*The American Negro,* by Thomas, himself a coloured man).

INDEX

275

Index

Index

Index

Index

Index

Index

281

Index

O

OATHS—
    Chuka, 199
    Ngondu, 198
Old women as narrators of stories, 209
Ordeals—
    Akamba, 196
    Akikuyu, 196
    Heated knife, 61, 196
Original population, 20-24

P

PHYSICAL characteristics of the Chuka, 42
"Picture gourds," 166
Pigott, Mr, Acting District Commissioner, 235
Pipes, Chuka, 129
Pitfalls, 155
Pith-hat dance, 174
"Plantain birds," 21
Poison for arrows, 156
Polygamy, 71
Population of Kenya, 20
Potatoes, 102
Pottery, 133
Pottery nozzle a potent charm, 131
Prostitution, 71
Psychology of the crowd, 258
Punishment, 270

Q

QUIVERS, 157

R

RAIDS, 159
    On the Chuka, 30, 31
Rain incantations, 201
Rape, 71
Religion, 205
    Christianity and Islam, 206, 264
    Sacred groves, 205
Renda dance, 176
Research, wide field for, 256
Riddles, 221-226
Rinderpest, 117
Rivers of Kenya, 23
Roman Catholic Mission, 37
Rukwara strap, the, 83, 86
Rupingazi river, 31

S

SACRED groves, 205
Salt, 97, 103
Sanitation, 112, 116
Seduction, 70
Sensibility and perception of the negro, 44
Shaving the head, 92, 137
Sheath, sword, 147
Shields, 119, 157
    Bark, 158
    Chuka, 158
    Dance, 158
    Mkongoro, the, 158
Singing, 168
Skins, the working of, 131
Slave raider, influence of the, 38
Smithy, a native, 129
Snuff, 128

Index

Index

W

WANDEROBO, the, 21
  Trap for animals, 123
War, the effect of the Great, on the native, 271
Warfare, 159
  Organization, 160
  Raids, 159
  Renda dance, 161
  Truce, 160
  Women in, 160
Weapons—
  Axes, 149
  Bow, 142
  Bows and arrows, 151
  Clubs, 149
  Defence, 157
  Masai warrior, 146
  Mkongoro, 158
  Offence, 143
  Poison, 156

Weapons—*cont.*
  Quiver, 157
  Shield, 157
  Spear, 142
  Wizard's bow, 155
Weapons, Masai influence, 141
White travellers, slight influence of, 37
Wilson, Sir R. K., 62*n.*
Wire-work, 164
Witch-doctor, the, 183
Wives, faithfulness of, 71
Wizard, the, in the Elders' Councils, 56
Wizard's bow, 155
Women—
  Conservatism of, 267
  In connection with land tenure, 65
  Petticoats of, 138
  Physical characteristics of, 46, 47

284

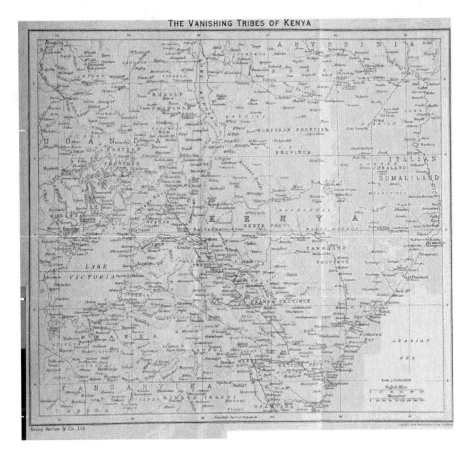

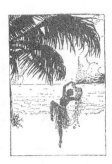
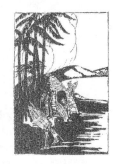
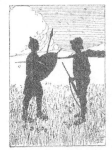
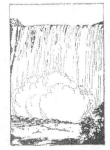

SPORT & WILD LIFE IN THE DECCAN.

AN ACCOUNT OF BIG-GAME HUNTING DURING OVER THIRTY YEARS OF SERVICE IN INDIA, WITH MUCH INTERESTING INFORMATION OF THE HABITS OF WILD ANIMALS OF THAT COUNTRY. By Brig.-Gen. R. G. BURTON, Author of "History of the Hyderabad Contingent," Wellington's Campaigns in India," &c. &c. With Illustrations & Map. 21s. nett.

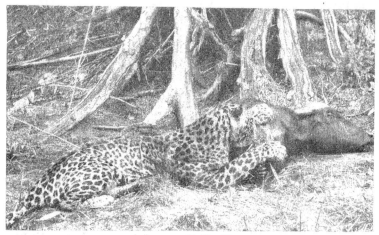

A LEOPARD & HIS KILL.

WANDERINGS IN CENTRAL AFRICA.

THE EXPERIENCES & ADVENTURES OF A LIFETIME OF PIONEERING & EXPLORATION. By DUGALD CAMPBELL, F.R.G.S., F.R.A.I., Author of "On the Trail of the Veiled Tuareg." With Illustrations & Map. Demy 8vo. 21s. nett.

THE LAND PIRATES OF INDIA. AN ACCOUNT

OF THE KURAVERS, A REMARKABLE TRIBE OF HEREDITARY CRIMINALS, THEIR EXTRAORDINARY SKILL AS THIEVES, CATTLE-LIFTERS, & HIGH-WAYMEN, &c., AND THEIR MANNERS & CUSTOMS. By W. J. HATCH. With Illustrations & Map. 21s. nett.

SEELEY, SERVICE & CO. LTD., 196 SHAFTESBURY AVENUE, W.C. 2

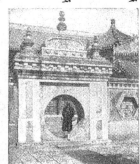

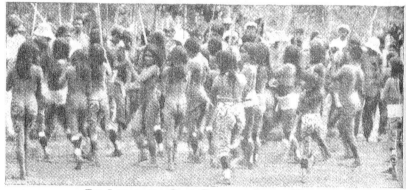

IN UNKNOWN NEW GUINEA. A RECORD OF

TWENTY-FIVE YEARS OF PERSONAL OBSERVATION & EXPERIENCE AMONGST THE INTERESTING PEOPLE OF A HITHERTO UNKNOWN PART OF THIS VAST ISLAND, & A DESCRIPTION OF THEIR MANNERS & CUSTOMS, OCCUPATIONS IN PEACE & METHODS OF WARFARE, THEIR SECRET RITES & PUBLIC CEREMONIES. By W. J. V. SAVILLE. With Introduction by B. MALINOWSKI, Ph.D., D.Sc., Lecturer in Social Anthropology, London University. With 58 Illustrations & Maps. 21s. nett. ✄ ✄

"Every detail of life among these savage peoples, including their secret ceremonies, is described with accuracy and often with vivid power."—*The Spectator.*

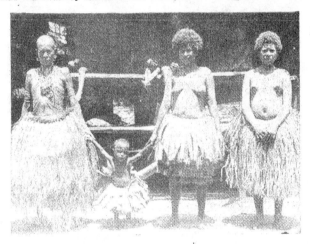

NATIVE WOMEN'S SKIRTS.
1. A widow's. 2. A baby girl's first. 3. A best dress. 4. A workaday dress.

ROD FISHING in NEW ZEALAND WATERS.

A DESCRIPTION OF A FISHERMAN'S PARADISE WITH ITS TEEMING LAKES, RIVERS & SEAS, THE STORY OF THE INTRODUCTION OF GAME FISH, & FULL INFORMATION ABOUT SPORT, EQUIPMENT, REGULATIONS & CAMPING. By T. E. DONNE, C.M.G. With Illustrations & Map. 12s. 6d. nett.

✄ ✄ ✄

ARABS IN TENT & TOWN. AN INTIMATE

ACCOUNT OF THE FAMILY LIFE OF THE ARABS OF SYRIA, THEIR MANNER OF LIVING IN DESERT & TOWN, THEIR HOSPITALITY, CUSTOMS, & MENTAL ATTITUDE, WITH A DESCRIPTION OF THE ANIMALS, BIRDS, FLOWERS & PLANTS OF THEIR COUNTRY. By A. GOODRICH-FREER, F.R.S.G.S., Author of "Things Seen in Palestine," "In a Syrian Saddle," &c. &c. With many Illustrations. 21s. nett. ✄ ✄

"An extremely good book of a rather unusual kind."—*Birmingham Post.*

"Throughout this large volume there is not a single dull line. One of the most attractive travel books of the year."—*The Lady.*

SEELEY, SERVICE & CO. LTD., 196 SHAFTESBURY AVENUE, W.C. 2

THE THINGS SEEN SERIES

Each Volume profusely illustrated.   Cloth, 3s. 6d. net ; Leather, 5s. net.

"A successful series by capable writers."—*The Times.*

"Beautifully illustrated with photographs of characteristic scenes and people."—*The Daily Telegraph.*

"As each new volume of 'Things Seen' comes out it serves to show how admirably the whole series has been planned & how capably the work has been carried out. The little books have a character & quality of their own."—*British Weekly,* Dec, 10th, '25.

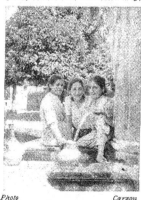

Photo   Carzon

Women at the Fountain, Cordova.

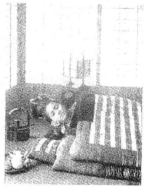

Stereo Copyright   Underwood & U.
London & N. York.

Geisha asleep between wadded quilts.

Complete List of Volumes in the Series.

Things Seen in

JAPAN. Clive Holland.
N. INDIA. T. L. Pennell.
CHINA. J. R. Chitty.
HOLLAND. C. E. Roche.
FLORENCE. E. Grierson.
CONSTANTINOPLE. Mrs. Spoer.
PALESTINE. A. Goodrich-Freer.
VENICE. L. M Ragg.
SWEDEN. W. B. Steveni.
EGYPT. E. L. Butcher.
ITALIAN LAKES. L. Ragg.
EDINBURGH. E. Grierson.
PARIS. Clive Holland.

OXFORD. N. J. Davidson.
SPAIN. C. G. Hartley.
LONDON. A. H. Blake, M.A.
RIVIERA. Capt. Richardson.
SWITZERLAND [Winter] Fife.
ENGLISH LAKES. W.T.Palmer.
ROME. A. G. Mackinnon, M.A.
NORWAY. S. C. Hammer, M.A.
CANADA. J. E. Ray.
SWITZERLAND [Summer]Ashby.
NORMANDY & BRITTANY,
SHAKESPEARE'S COUNTRY.
Clive Holland.

PYRENEES. Capt. Richardson.
NORTH WALES. W. T. Palmer.
TOWER OF LONDON.
H. Plunket Woodgate.
BAY OF NAPLES. Including
Pompei, Naples, Sorrento,
Amalfi, Capri, &c. &c.
A. G. Mackinnon.
MADEIRA. J. E. Hutcheon.
DOLOMITES. L. M. Davidson.
PROVENCE. Capt. Richardson.
MOROCCO. L. E. Bickerstaffe,
M.A.

SEELEY'S TRAVEL BOOKS GEOGRAPHICALLY GROUPED

AFRICA

AFRICAN IDYLLS. The Right Rev. Donald Fraser, D.D. 6s. nett.
AMONG BANTU NOMADS. J. Tom Brown. 21s.
AMONG THE PRIMITIVE BAKONGO. John H. Weeks. 16s. nett.
A CAMERA ACTRESS IN AFRICAN WILDS. M. Gehrts. 12s. 6d. nett.
A NATURALIST IN MADAGASCAR. James Sibree, LL.D., F.R.G.S. 16s. nett.
CAMP & TRAMP IN AFRICAN WILDS. E. Torday. 16s. nett.
FIGHTING THE SLAVE HUNTERS IN CENTRAL AFRICA. A. J. Swann. 16s. nett.
IN ASHANTI & BEYOND. A. W. Cardinall, F.R.G.S., F.R.A.I. 21s. nett.
IN THE HEART OF BANTULAND. D. Campbell. 21s. nett.
IN WITCH-BOUND AFRICA. Frank H. Melland, B.A., F.R.A.I., F.R.G.S., F.Z.S. 21s nett
MYSTERIES OF THE LIBYAN DESERT. W. J. Harding King, F.R.G.S. 21s. nett.
THE LIFE & EXPLORATIONS OF F. S. ARNOT. Rev. E. Baker. 12s. 6d. & 6s. nett.
ON THE TRAIL OF THE BUSHONGO. E. Torday, F.R.A.S. 21s. nett.
ON THE TRAIL OF THE VEILED TUAREG. Dugald Campbell, F.R.A.I. 21s. nett.
PYGMIES & BUSHMEN OF THE KALAHARI. S. S. Dornan, F.R.A.I., F.R.G.S. 21s. nett.
RIFT VALLEYS & GEOLOGY OF EAST AFRICA. Prof. J. W. Gregory, F.R.S., D.SC. 32s. nett.
SAVAGE LIFE IN THE BLACK SUDAN. C. W. Domville-Fife. 21s. nett.
SPORT & ADVENTURE IN AFRICA. Capt. T. W. Shorthose. 21s. nett.
SPORT & SERVICE IN AFRICA. Lieut.-Col. A. H. W. Haywood, C.M.G., D.S.O. 21s. nett.

AFRICA—*continued.*

To the Mysterious Lorian Swamp. Capt. C. Wightwick Haywood. 21s. nett.
The Autobiography of an African. Donald Fraser, D.D. 6s. nett.
The Cliff Dwellers of Kenya. J. A. Massam. 21s. nett.
The Spirit-ridden Konde. D. R. MacKenzie, F.R.G.S. 21s. nett.
Through Jubaland to the Lorian Swamp. I. N. Dracopoli, F.R.G.S. 16s. nett.
Unconquered Abyssinia as it is To-day. Charles F. Rey, F.R.G.S. 21s. nett. [16s. nett.
Vanishing Tribes of Kenya. Major G. St. J. Orde Brown, O.B.E., F.R.G.S., F.R.A.I., F.Z.S.
Wanderings in Central Africa. Dugald Campbell, F.R.G.S. 21s. nett.
Wild Bush Tribes of Tropical Africa. G. Cyril Claridge. 21s. nett.

ASIA

A Diplomat in Japan. Sir Ernest Satow, G.C.M.G. 32s. nett. [6s. nett.
Among the Wild Tribes of the Afghan Frontier. T. L. Pennell, M.D., F.R.C.S. 16s. &
Among Primitive Peoples in Borneo. Ivor H. N. Evans, B.A. 21s. nett.
A Burmese Arcady. Major C. M. Enriquez, F.R.G.S. 21s. nett.
Arabs in Tent & Town. A. Goodrich-Freer, F.R.S.G.S. 21s. nett.
In Farthest Burma. Capt. F. Kingdon Ward. 25s. nett. [B.SC. 21s. nett.
In Himalayan Tibet. Reeve Heber, M.D., CH.B., & Kathleen M. Heber, M.B., CH.B.,
In the Nicobar Islands. George Whitehead, B.A. 21s. nett.
In Unknown China. S. Pollard. 25s. nett.
Kashmir in Sunlight & Shade. C. E. Tyndale-Biscoe, M.A. 6s. nett.
Land Pirates of India. W. J. Hatch. 21s. nett.
A Military Consul in Turkey. Capt. A. F. Townshend. 16s. nett.
Magic Ladakh. "Ganpat" (Major L. M. A. Gompertz). 21s. nett.
Mystery Rivers of Tibet. Capt. F. Kingdon Ward, B.A., F.R.G.S. 21s. nett.
Pennell of the Afghan Frontier. A. M. Pennell, M.B., B.S.(Lond.), B.SC. 6s. nett.
Persian Women & Their Ways. C. Colliver Rice. 21s. nett.
Romantic Java: As It Was & Is. Hubert S. Banner, B.A., F.R.G.S. 21s. nett.
Sea Gypsies of Malaya. W. C. White, M.A. 21s. nett.
The Making of Modern Japan. John H. Gubbins, M.A.(Oxon), C.M.G. 21s. nett.
Through Kamchatka by Dog-Sled & Skis. Sten Bergman, D.SC. 21s. nett.
Through Khiva to Golden Samarkand. E. Christie, F.R.G.S. 21s. nett. [25s. nett.
To the Alps of Chinese Tibet. Prof. J. W. Gregory, F.R.S., D.SC., & C. J. Gregory, B.SC.
Two Gentlemen of China. Lady Hosie. 21s. & 7s. 6d. nett.
Sport & Wild Life in the Deccan. Brig.-Gen. R. G. Burton. 21s. nett.
We Tibetans. Rin-Chen Lha-Mo. 12s. 6d. nett.

AMERICA

Among the Eskimos of Labrador. S. K. Hutton, M.B. 16s. nett.
Among Wild Tribes of the Amazons. C. W. Domville-Fife. 21s. nett.
A Church in the Wilds. W. Barbrooke Grubb. 6s. nett.
An Unknown People in an Unknown Land. W. Barbrooke Grubb. 16s. & 6s. nett.
Mexico in Revolution. C. Cameron, O.B.E., F.R.G.S. 21s. nett.

AUSTRALASIA

Among Papuan Headhunters. E. Baxter Riley, F.R.A.I. 21s. nett.
The Maori: Past & Present. T. E. Donne, C.M.G. 21s. nett.
Rod Fishing in New Zealand Waters. T. E. Donne, C.M.G. 12s. 6d. nett.
The Hill Tribes of Fiji. A. B. Brewster. 21s. nett.
In Primitive New Guinea. J. H. Holmes. 21s. nett.
In the Isles of King Solomon. A. I. Hopkins. 21s. nett.
In Unknown New Guinea. W. J. V. Saville. 21s. nett.
The Land of the New Guinea Pygmies. Lt.-Col. C. D. Rawling, C.I.E., F.R.G.S. 16s. n.
Unexplored New Guinea. Wilfred N. Beaver. 25s. nett.

OTHER PARTS OF THE WORLD

Among Unknown Eskimo. Julian W. Bilby. 21s. nett.
A Naturalist at the Poles. R. N. Rudmose Brown, D.SC. 25s. nett.
Enchanted Days with Rod and Gun. Captain Alban F. L. Bacon. 12s. 6d. nett.
Human Migration & the Future. Professor J. W. Gregory, F.R.S., D.SC. 12s. 6d. nett.
Memories of Four Continents. Lady Glover. 16s. nett.
Modern Whaling & Bear Hunting. W. G. Burn Murdoch. 25s. nett.
Modern Travel. Norman J. Davidson, B.A.(Oxon.). 25s. nett.
Spitzbergen. R. N. Rudmose Brown, D.SC. 25s. nett.
The Menace of Colour. Prof. J. W. Gregory, F.R.S., D.SC. 12s. 6d. nett.

Miscellanea

JUST PUBLISHED

THE ENGLISH BIBLE & ITS STORY.

ITS GROWTH, ITS TRANSLATORS & THEIR ADVENTURES. By JAMES BAIKIE, D.D., F.R.A.S., Author of "The Glamour of Near East Excavation," &c. With Illustrations. Demy 8vo. 10s. 6d. nett.

THE GLAMOUR OF NEAR EAST EXCAVATION. AN ACCOUNT OF THE TREASURE-HUNT FOR THE BURIED ART, WISDOM & HISTORY OF THE ANCIENT EAST, FROM THE NILE TO BABYLON, THE ADVENTURES, DISAPPOINTMENTS & TRIUMPHS OF THE HUNTERS, & THE KNOWLEDGE THUS ACQUIRED OF THE ANCIENT WORLD. By JAMES BAIKIE, F.R.A.S. Demy 8vo. Illustrated. 10s. 6d. nett.

SECOND EDITION

CROOKS & CRIME. DESCRIBING THE METHODS OF CRIMINALS FROM THE AREA SNEAK TO THE PROFESSIONAL CARD-SHARPER, FORGER, OR MURDERER, & THE VARIOUS WAYS IN WHICH THEY ARE CIRCUMVENTED & CAPTURED. By J. KENNETH FERRIER, formerly Scotland Yard, C.I.D. Detective Inspector. With Illustrations. 18s. nett.

HUMAN MIGRATION & THE FUTURE.

A STUDY OF THE CAUSES OF POPULATION MOVEMENTS, & THE IM-PORTANCE OF FACILITY OF TRANSFER OF SURPLUSES FROM CROWDED TO SPARSELY PEOPLED COUNTRIES. By Professor J. W. GREGORY, F.R.S., D.Sc., Professor of Geology in the University of Glasgow, Author of "The Menace of Colour," "The Rift Valleys & Geology of East Africa," "Geology of To-day," &c. With Illustrations. Demy 8vo. 12s. 6d. nett.

SECOND EDITION

THE MENACE OF COLOUR. A STUDY OF THE DIFFICULTIES DUE TO THE ASSOCIATION OF WHITE & COLOURED RACES, WITH AN ACCOUNT OF MEASURES PROPOSED FOR THEIR SOLUTION & SPECIAL REFERENCE TO WHITE COLONIZATION IN THE TROPICS. By Prof. J. W. GREGORY, F.R.S., D.Sc., Professor of Geology in the University of Glasgow, Author of "The Rift Valleys & Geology of East Africa," "The Great Rift Valley," "Geology of To-day," &c., and Co-Author of "To the Alps of Chinese Tibet." Demy 8vo. With Illustrations & Maps. 12s. 6d. nett.

"The handiest & most comprehensive statement of the colour question available. Professor Gregory's statements can be accepted without qualification."—*Review of Reviews.*

SEELEY, SERVICE & CO. LTD., 196 SHAFTESBURY AVENUE, W.C. 2

SEELEY'S NEW TRAVEL BOOKS, SPRING 1925

THE VANISHING TRIBES OF KENYA. A Description of the Manners & Customs of the Primitive & Interesting Tribes dwelling on the vast Southern Slopes of Mount Kenya, & their Fast-disappearing Native Methods of Life. By Major G. St. J. Orde Browne, O.B.E., F.R.G.S., F.R.A.I., F.Z.S. Late Royal Artillery, Senior Commissioner, Tanganyika. Many Illustrations & 2 Maps. 21s. nett.

MEXICO IN REVOLUTION. An Account of an Englishwoman's Experiences & Adventures in the Land of Revolution, with a Description of the People, the Beauties of the Country & the Highly Interesting Remains of Aztec Civilization. By Charlotte Cameron, O.B.E., F.R.G.S. Illustrations. 21s. nett.

ON THE TRAIL OF THE BUSHONGO. An Account of a Remarkable & Hitherto Unknown African People, their Origin, Art, High Social & Political Organization, & Culture, derived from the author's personal experience amongst them. By E. Torday. Member of the Council of the Royal Anthropological Institute of Great Britain; Corresponding Fellow of the Anthropological Society of Vienna. With 59 Illustrations & a Map. 21s. nett.

THE MENACE OF COLOUR. With Special Reference to White Colonization of the Tropics. By Professor J. W. Gregory, D.Sc., F.R.S., Professor of Geology in the University of Glasgow. Author of "To the Alps of Chinese Tibet," &c., &c. Illustrations & Maps. 12s. 6d. nett.

Books Issued Within the Last Twelve Months

FOURTH EDITION

TWO GENTLEMEN OF CHINA. An Intimate Description of the Private Life of Two Patrician Chinese Families. Lady Hosie. Illustrations. 21s.
"Nothing more intimate has been written on China."—*Nation.*

ARABS IN TENT & TOWN. By A. Goodrich-Freer, F.R.G.S. Many Illustrations. 21s. nett.
"A delightful & valuable book simply packed with fascinating detail."—*Daily M'l.*

TO THE ALPS OF CHINESE TIBET. J. W. Gregory, D.Sc., F.R.S. Illustrations & Maps. 25s. nett.
"High adventure."—*Manchester Guardian.*

A NATURALIST AT THE POLES. The Life, Work & Voyages of Dr. W. S. Bruce, the Polar Explorer. R. N. Rudmose Brown, D.Sc. Illustrations & 3 Maps. 25s. nett.
"This admirable Biography is worthy of Bruce."—*Westminster Gazette.*

IN WITCH-BOUND AFRICA. Frank H. Melland, B.A.(Oxon). Many Illustrations & a Map. 21s. nett.
"Extraordinarily fascinating and profoundly interesting."—*Birmingham Post.*

PYGMIES & BUSHMEN OF THE KALAHARI. By S. S. Dornan, F.R.G.S., F.R.A.I. Many Illustrations & a Map. 21s. nett.
"A fascinating book."—*Cork Examiner.*
"Of remarkable interest."
—*Newcastle Chronicle.*

THE MYSTERY RIVERS OF TIBET. Captain F. Kingdon Ward, B.A., F.R.G.S. Illustrations & 3 Maps. 21s. nett.
"One of the most puzzling and interesting sections of the earth's surface."
Scotsman.

SECOND EDITION

AMONG WILD TRIBES OF THE AMAZONS. By C. W. Domville-Fife. Illustrations & 6 Maps. 21s. nett.
"A most thrilling description of thrilling experiences."—*Saturday Review.*

IN THE NICOBAR ISLANDS. By George Whitehead, B.A. With a Preface by Sir Richard C. Temple, Bart., C.B., C.I.E. Many Illustrations & a Map. 21s. nett.
"Singularly vivid & interesting."
—*Birmingham Gazette.*

MEMORIES OF FOUR CONTINENTS. Lady Glover. 16s. nett.
"Abounds in good stories."
Northern Whig.

UNCONQUERED ABYSSINIA As It Is To-day. Charles F. Rey, F.R.G.S. Illustrations. 21s. nett.
"Mr. Rey lifts the veil hanging over Abyssinia."—*Morning Post.*

AMONG UNKNOWN ESKIMO. Julian W. Bilby, F.R.G.S. With Illustrations & 2 Maps. 21s. nett.
"This interesting, indeed absorbing volume."—*Aberdeen Journal.*

SPORT & ADVENTURE IN AFRICA. Captain T. W. Shorthose, D.S.O. Illustrations & a Map. 21s. nett.
"Vies with Selous, Cotton, Oswell, and Gordon-Cumming."—*Scotsman.*

THE AUTOBIOGRAPHY OF AN AFRICAN. The Life Story of an African Chief. By Donald Fraser, D.D. With Illustrations. 6s. nett.
"Unique. . . . Missionary work as seen through the native eye and mind. . . . The central figure, a chief's warrior son, will rejoice many readers of Rider Haggard."
Review of Reviews.

THIRD EDITION

AFRICAN IDYLLS. Donald Fraser, D.D. With Illustrations. 6s. nett.
"Bears the stamp of genius."—*Scotsman.*

SEELEY, SERVICE & CO. LIMITED.

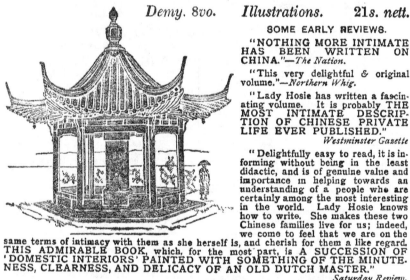

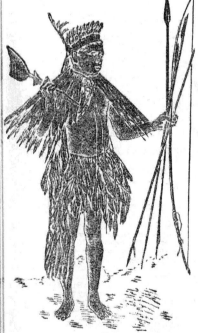

SPORT & ADVENTURE
IN AFRICA

A Record of Twelve Years of Big Game Hunting Campaigning & Travel in the Wilds of Tropical Africa

BY

CAPTAIN W. T. SHORTHOSE, D.S.O.,
F.R.G.S., F.R.A.I., F.Z.S.

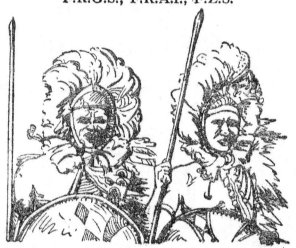

WARUSHA MORAN WARRIORS IN FIGHTING KIT.

With Many Illustrations & a Map.   *Demy 8vo.*   *21s. nett.*

SOME EARLY REVIEWS.

"Captain Shorthose is a sportsman-traveller-soldier of keen observation and wide interests. He gives us details of elephant, rhinoceros, hippopotamus and buffalo shooting and some striking adventures. VIES WITH THE WORKS OF F. C. SELOUS, COTTON OSWELL AND ROUALEYN GORDON-CUMMING."—*The Scotsman.*

"Another of the admirable books of travel and sport in which Messrs. Seeley, Service & Co. specialise. . . . The author enjoys excitement, and enables us to enjoy it as he goes out to meet some of the most dangerous animals."—*Daily News.*

"The book, WELL ILLUSTRATED FROM VERY UNIQUE PHOTOGRAPHS and packed with epic adventures, is the racy record of a full twelve years in the life of an observant, impressionable explorer and soldier."—*Western Daily Press.*

"The book is A CHEERY, ENTERTAINING, PERSONAL NARRATIVE, unpretentious, and yet quite capably written. It will be thoroughly enjoyed by that large circle of Englishmen which enjoys hearing a plain narrative of exciting adventures."
Birmingham Post.

"Captain Shorthose tells many strange, true travellers' tales in the volume and tells them well. . . . FULL OF EXCITING AND VARIED EXPERIENCES. . . . HE IS A MIGHTY HUNTER."—*Northern Whig.*

"A record of twelve years of big game hunting, campaigning and travels in the wilds of Africa, all graphically written, and full of exciting incidents and quaint experiences."
Naval and Military Record.

"Captain W. T. Shorthose, D.S.O., narrates an exciting fight with an elephant—in which the elephant nearly won—in AN EXCELLENT BOOK OF TRAVEL. The book is a noteworthy addition to the publishers' great library of travel stories."—*Daily Graphic.*

"The author, as becomes a successful hunter, is a keen observer of country, tribes and their ways, and wild beasts and their haunts. In addition he is gifted with a facile pen which immediately grips the reader's attention until his story is told."
Sheffield Daily Telegraph.

SEELEY, SERVICE & CO., 196 SHAFTESBURY AVENUE, W.C.2

CPSIA information can be obtained
at www.ICGtesting.com
Printed in the USA
BVHW050003140223
658390BV00008B/204